Clinical Audit for Nurses and Therapists

Clinical Audit for Nurses and Therapists

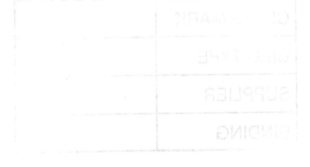

Rebecca Malby RN, DipN, MA
Director of Nursing Practice
The Institute of Nursing
The University of Leeds

with 5 contributors

Scutari Press
London

First published 1995
Reprinted 1995

British Library Cataloguing in Publication Data
Malby, Rebecca
Clinical Audit for Nurses and Therapists
I. Title
362.110941

ISBN 1–873853–09–2

Typeset by J&L Composition Ltd, Filey, North Yorkshire
Printed and bound by Bell and Bain Ltd., Glasgow

Contents

Contributors

Haydn Cook MA MHSM DipHSM
Chief Executive, Northallerton Health Services NHS Trust

Rebecca Malby RN DipN MA
Director, Nursing Practice, Institute of Nursing, Leeds University

Jan Maycock RGN RM
Assistant Director, Institute of Nursing, Leeds University

Cathy McCargow RN RM HV MBA
Nurse Adviser, Leicester Health Authority

Christine Payne MSc DANS RGN RCNT DipN(Lond)
Director of Nursing and Quality, Dartford and Gravesend Acute Unit

Deborah Wheeler BSc(Hons) RGN OnC DipN
Senior Nurse/Business Manager, Royal National Orthopaedic Hospital
NHS Trust

Preface

Audit has become the latest buzzword within the NHS. It brings with it the fear of change and the feeling of riding a camel in the desert without a guide. The attendance at audit conferences is phenomenal as newly appointed audit officers attempt to make sense of the process and look for solutions to their difficulties. In this book I do not provide quick fix solutions to audit; there are none, despite many claims to the contrary. Rather, I attempt to explore the reasons why audit is successful, or unsuccessful, and offer approaches based on experience and organisational analysis that the reader may find helpful.

I first became interested in audit when helping to set up a nursing development unit. At that time we wanted to show that we could improve care and provide value for money. We wanted to demonstrate the valuable contribution that nursing makes to patient outcomes and efficient and effective services. What emerged from that experience was that the service in which we work is fraught with overt and hidden agendas, with professional territorialism, and with little understanding of how to actively engage the client in improving treatment and care. This culture provides the backdrop to any challenges or attempts at change and, therefore, to the completion of the audit cycle. This book explores that culture and options for ways forward. I have also attempted to pick up the crystal ball and predict the future for audit. It is anticipated that the reader will dip in and out of some sections of the book, picking relevant and helpful sections as necessary. Some topics will, therefore, be covered from different angles (e.g. quality).

The therapy professions have been the Cinderellas of audit (as with many initiatives). I have attempted to reflect their position, recognising their unique skills and the opportunities for measuring outcomes that are afforded to them. Undoubtedly, though, their current stage of development in relation to audit is mirrored in the book. I would be delighted to include a chapter specific to therapy audit in a future edition.

Throughout the book I have used the terms client and patient interchangeably. Readers are asked to interpret this as they feel most relevant to their own settings.

Rebecca Malby

1

The Whys and Wherefores of Audit

Introduction

Audit is a confusing term. To the lay person it brings to mind accountants poring over 'the books' to seek out any errant financial practices. Most people's relationship with their auditor is a mixture of regard, apprehension and defensiveness and the outcome of the audit is usually tinged with feelings of relief. The use of the term 'audit' in the NHS usually refers to a centrally-driven initiative to introduce systematic analysis of clinical practices. This type of audit has some similarities to financial audit with which we are familiar:

- It involves scrutiny of current and past practices.
- It involves comparisons of actual practices with agreed standards.
- It examines these practices to see if the best use was made of resources.
- It brings on a feeling of defensiveness in those being audited.

So how did the concept of audit come to feature so centrally in the running of the NHS? How has it emerged to attract such significant resources? Is audit a passing phase or is it here to stay? Equally important as those questions that probe into the purpose of audit are the questions: How do you actually carry out audit and make it work? What are the pitfalls? How does audit fit into the many other priorities that seem to be bombarding the NHS at the moment?

This book seeks to answer these questions in relation to the nursing and therapy professions. This chapter will take us from the conception of audit within the NHS to the present day. In attempting to put audit into a political framework, the chapter will identify the tensions underlying medical audit, the difficulties in moving into clinical audit, and the ways that clinical audit can learn the lessons of the past to determine its future.

The differences between medical audit and nursing and therapy audit

Many texts and articles have been written about medical audit, and considering the resources that it has attracted, this is hardly surprising. However, the patient's experience of clinical care and the service as a whole goes far beyond the interventions of one professional group. Nurses and therapists have achieved significant success in changing practices as part of the audit cycle. These changes are rarely within the domain of their own discrete professional boundaries; they have sought to collaborate in advancing all aspects of the patient's experience. The different approach that nurses and therapists have taken from medical audit stems from several factors:

- The fact that nursing and therapy theory has a social science base as well as a positivist biomedical base. This means that they are more familiar with evaluative research and the use of questionnaires and interviews. While audit is not research, much of the data collection relies on research tools. Moreover, social sciences tend not to take a purely positivist approach (i.e. hypothesis testing), rather, they are open to development of ideas in relation to the human factors that contribute to situations. This makes nurses and therapists more comfortable with the process of audit.
- The fact that nurses primarily have a track record in the setting of standards and thus a literature base to this activity (Kitson, 1989). There has been a trend in nursing to develop a 'bottom up' approach to standards. Nurses are taught standard setting, and will have experience in developing their own standards. The difficulty with standard setting in the nursing arena is the lack of definitive research in some areas on which to base the standard. This is not a trend mirrored in medicine. The Donabedian approach to standards is just hitting the medical press. To date standards in medicine have tended to mean protocols.
- The fact that nurses play a strong coordinating role in the provision of a holistic service to the patient. This means that nurses in particular are used to planning their care alongside their professional colleagues, and have access on a regular basis to all members of the multidisciplinary team. Nurses are likely to be particularly familiar with the organisational elements of the service that hinder care delivery (such as poor communication, cross-boundary misunderstanding, the effects of one profession's decision on the rest of the team).
- The fact that nursing and therapy interventions are directed at goal attainment. Nurses, through care planning, and therapists, through problem-orientated records, have developed a recording system that anticipates expected goals, negotiates these with the patient, and evalu-

ates achievement against these goals. Therapists are also developing scoring mechanisms for evaluating their interventions. Medical notes tend to be a descriptive dialogue about the pattern of events. Thus nurses and therapists have the beginnings of a framework for outcome measurement.

- The fact that nurses and therapists are managed within the general management system and gave up their recourse to professional line management long ago. Nurses and therapists are used to having their performance evaluated by managers outside their profession. They have thus begun to tackle the issues of accountability and professional autonomy and are relatively used to presenting their performance in a format meaningful to managers, and involving them in that evaluation process. Thus the sensitivities around the scrutiny of professional practice by other health care staff, while not being completely overcome, have been worked through to a greater extent than in medicine. In other words, at the current state of play, doctors perceive they have more to lose in sharing any evaluation of their professional performance through audit.

- The fact that nurses, and to a lesser extent therapists, have been the target for cost improvement exercises largely through skill mix studies with the explicit end point of cost reduction. Nurses in particular, as the largest proportion of the NHS pay expenditure, are usually the first port of call for any cost reduction exercises. This is coupled with an increasing emphasis on the attainment of task based competencies that go to make up vocational qualifications in an attempt to bring the pay bill down, and to de-professionalise nursing activity. Therapists too have been under the microscope to determine the extent to which the health service requires so many different professional groups. These skill mix studies have brought to the fore the question of the value for money of professional practice, with conflicting results. Thus nurses and therapists have been exposed to the necessity to explain and demonstrate the value they bring as experts and professionals. Medicine is unlikely to face the same detailed scrutiny but it is inevitable, with the increases in demand for the service and the necessity to contain cost, that medicine will not walk free without a certain degree of frisking first.

Nurses and therapists have been subject to external and internal scrutiny, have been closely tied into quality initiatives, and have been developing methods to evaluate their practices. Doctors, on the other hand, have been spared the close managerial scrutiny of their practices, though this looks set to change. Due to the nature of the work they do (i.e. treatment) they have a stronger research literature on the best treatment to use in a given situation. Doctors' rewards (i.e. promotion and merit awards) are related primarily to research and publication and thus 'expertise', rather than ability to deliver a value for money service. Medicine has a different research base (both financial and theoretical) and different concerns when it comes to any review of that practice. These different backgrounds serve to bring into relief the difficulties that we will, and do, have in bringing the professions together to undertake clinical audit. The importance of history and context in the development of clinical audit cannot be under-represented. In order to describe the answers to the practical question of how, I need to take you on a trip down memory lane to the inception of the NHS reforms.

Working for patients

The internal market was first proposed by Enthoven (1985), introducing limited competition to overcome the 'perverse incentives' which he thought constrained good management and clinical ability in a centrally planned and managed public sector. The introduction of an 'internal market' and the division of purchaser and provider roles came into effect on 1 April 1991, as a result of the NHS Act 1990 which followed the White Paper *Working for Patients* (1989a). The reorganisation was the latest of government attempts to improve efficiency and control cost, while optimising the effectiveness of the service. It centred around the internal market, in which hospitals and community services compete for contracts. The purchasers of the service, with whom contracts are placed on behalf of the patient, are GP fundholders, district health authorities (DHAs) and FHSAs, and private sources. The intention was to retain universal access to the service, while increasing consumer choice and improving value for money.

Another element of the reforms was the widespread introduction of mandatory medical audit. These key areas reflected a long-standing drive by the government to focus managerial activity on the provision of a service that could be demonstrated as value for money. Previous initiatives to improve performance included management budgeting, resource management and performance indicators. Medical audit was seen by policy makers as a way of calling doctors to account for their practices by drawing them into performance measurement within the new NHS market. Previous attempts to bring doctors into a managerial structure that made them at least accountable for their resources (as clinical directors within resource management sites), had achieved only a small degree of success (Packwood *et al*, 1991). The sensitivity of this move to medical audit meant that few policy makers were willing to come clean on their motives. Thus doctors led by the Royal Colleges persisted with the belief that they had won a major initiative to advance medical practice through peer review and education. These mixed messages put medical audit on an unsteady footing from the start.

Moreover the *medical* audit initiative was just that. It directed resources and importance to only one section of a patient's clinical experience – the doctor's contribution. Nurses and therapists expressed great concern that large sums of public sector money were being directed at only one profession when many professions require tools to improve their practice and contribute to the patient's total experience of the health service. Indeed, in many instances, particularly in the community, the service given is predominantly that of nursing, and for some diagnoses, the major contributor to the patient's health gain is the therapist. One year after the instigation of medical audit, the nursing and therapy audit initiative was announced. The purpose was to ensure the development of a framework for nursing and therapy audit in all provider units. While the funding was significantly smaller than that available for medical audit, it meant that nurses and therapists had a resource to develop their own expertise in audit and to contribute to audit that crossed professional boundaries. Two years on, we are seeing the inception of clinical (multidisciplinary) audit. This reflects the fact that while all the professions required resources for unidisciplinary audit, there was a great deal of support for clinical audit. Much of the money went into projects that moved from unidisciplinary to multidisciplinary audit. At the same time, some medical audit committees widened their membership to include other professions, and used medical audit funding to support clinical audit projects. However, it must be noted that the major resource is still directed at medical audit, and that clinical audit funding for 1993/94 comes largely from underspends in the medical audit budget.

What is audit?

Audit is described as a cycle of activity (Tugwell and Mongonelli, 1986; see Figure 1.1). This cycle involves systematic review of practice, identification of problems, development of possible solutions, implementation of change, and then review again. Audit is essentially a form of peer review. Shaw (1990) has written extensively on the process of medical audit and suggests that it differs from traditional medical review by the fact that it uses measurements rather than judgements; it compares, numerically, current practices; practice is subjected to peer review; action to resolve discrepancies is identified; and, finally, the process is recorded in order to inform future management of cases. He argues that:

> . . . an effective system of audit contains three elements: agreed criteria for 'good' practice; methods of measuring performance against these criteria; and mechanisms for implementing appropriate change in practice.

Agreement on criteria for 'good' practice leads quite naturally to the establishment of clinical protocols for particular medical diagnosis, or

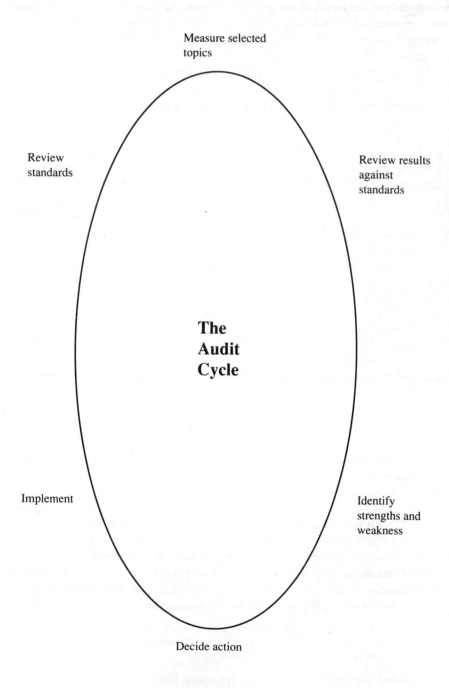

Figure 1.1 The audit cycle

standards for universal practices (e.g. discharge planning, IVI administration, referrals).

Nursing audit is defined as:

> . . . part of the cycle of quality assurance. It incorporates the systematic and critical analysis by nurses, midwives and health visitors, in conjunction with other staff, of the planning, delivery and evaluation of nursing and midwifery care, in terms of their use of resources and the outcomes for patients/clients, and introduces appropriate change in response to that analysis. (NHS ME, 1991. *Framework of Audit For Nursing Services*)

Nursing audit in this context is defined as the systematic evaluation of nursing resulting in improvements in the quality of care. The audit cycle involves measurement, review of practice, implementation of changes and re-measurement.

It is not surprising to see that, as with many 'new' discoveries in nursing, Florence Nightingale got there first. In 1863 she observed:

> In attempting to arrive at the truth, I have applied everywhere for information, but in scarcely an instance have I been able to obtain hospital records fit for any purpose of comparison. If they could be obtained they would enable us to decide many other questions beside the one alluded to. They would show subscribers how their money was being spent, what amount of good was really done with it, or whether the money was not doing mischief rather than good.

This identifies the central importance of service evaluation and the requirement for robust information to support it. Information is collected in the measurement phase of the cycle. To date in medical audit, the measurement phase has included both concurrent and retrospective audit. The latter requires the investigation of patient records after discharge to scrutinise the care actually received by the patient and its effects. The former includes the measurement of ongoing indices. Occurrence screening, or the monitoring of adverse patient occurrences, has been used in Brighton by Stevens and Bennett (1989). Criterion-based audit involves the selection of a topic for review (diagnosis, investigation, symptom), and criteria for reviewing the patient records (Shaw, 1990).

Medical audit appears to have been developing through three separate stages, namely:

1. Retrospective case note review   A particular clinical problem is identified by clinicians in discussion and casenotes are selected and searched to elicit the rate of occurrence and possible reasons behind it.

2. Criterion-based   Standards of clinical practice, relating for example to a particular disease, are discussed, defined and agreed. Instruments to monitor adherence to standards are developed. Patients are followed prospectively to determine adherence to agreed standards. After an agreed period (commonly 6–12 months) case notes and instruments are reviewed and discussed. Standards may be modified and clinical decisions clarified.

Alogorithm-based   A more sophisticated form of criterion audit which tries to describe the way in which treatment strategies are determined. For example:

Defining the flow of information about patients and the routes it follows.
Describing the diagnostic or therapeutic alogorithms and the weighting factors.
Considering trade-offs between alternatives.
Describing the roles of different agencies in the treatment process.

3. Outcome   This type of audit not only tries to define the question 'who does what to whom?', but also asks the more fundamental question 'did it do any good?' It makes the assumption that clinical research has shown that the treatments provided are effective. As purchasers move towards a health needs model to determine service provision the questions become:

How much did the patient benefit?
Do some patients benefit more than others?
What distinguishes between those who benefit most/least?
Where (ward, department, hospital) does the patient get the most effective and appropriate care?

Thus different kinds of information are required to answer these questions. These are:

(i)   Comprehensive measures of patient's health status before intervention and probably on several occasions after intervention.
(ii) Quantitative and qualitative measures of the treatment delivered and patient's perspective of these.
(iii) The costs of the treatment/care – economic and opportunity.

The importance of and interest in outcomes in the health service have led to the establishment of the National Clinical Outcomes Clearing House at the Nuffield Institute, University of Leeds, which seeks to document the viability of different health outcome measures. To date, outcome measures have concentrated primarily on quality of life indices.

Nursing and therapy audit has not been through the same development process but has undoubtedly been influenced by those methodologies used in medical audit. It has also been influenced by nurses' involvement in quality assurance and the national drive in nursing towards standard setting. In the therapy professions, audit has been influenced by the rise in problem-orientated records and the therapists' skills in functional assessment. The different methods for the audit cycle used within clinical audit are identified in more detail in Chapter 3.

The history of clinical audit

Evaluation in the public sector

Audit is the latest example of a drive in social policy over the last decade towards evaluation, particularly in the area of assessment of performance (Pollitt, 1986). This has pervaded the civil service, education, defence, the police and health. Roberts (1991) proposes that the reasons for being interested in the performance of the health service are clear

> . . . to establish in aggregate whether we are getting value for expenditure on health services and whether those services are effective.

Klein (1989) suggests that the government has been frustrated in its quest to determine how to monitor and assess the performance of a service, because it was unsure of how and to whom that service was being delivered. In other words, it believed it was being asked by the health service to write a blank cheque without knowing how long it would last or what it would be spent on. One initiative to overcome this frustration has been the development of performance indicators (clinical, managerial and estate management) (Pollitt, 1984) first issued in 1983, to be used in the new culture of managerial accountability. These indicators were a response to the belief that productivity could be improved through improved performance, within financial expediency. Most NHS performance indicators (PIs) were proxies for efficiency, only a few were for effectiveness or quality. Thus we saw the emergence of the precursors to league tables, much discussed these days in the field of education. The major criticism of PIs is that if you were performing within the middle range for a given activity, there was little incentive to improve. If you were at the bottom of the table, this could be due to circumstances beyond your control (i.e. the demographic nature of your population), meaning that you were in a no win situation. Being at the top of the table could likewise be circumstantial and might not reflect your managerial ability as, in reality, it could be possible for you to do a lot better. In other words, the indicators sought to over-simplify the performance of a complex service.

This quest for performance measurement materialised again in NHS reforms enshrined in the White Paper *Working for Patients*, in the form of medical audit and the introduction of the internal market. The internal market sought to produce incentives linked to productivity, price and quality of service. By using these three measures as indicators for the service and by removing purchasing of those services to another body, it was believed that the contracting process would wheedle out poor performers and encourage them to improve or suffer the consequences. Medical audit was seen as a way of at last evaluating doctors' performance in a way that contributed to the contracting process. To date, details or morbidity and mortality had been unavailable to consumers or their proxies (i.e. GP fundholders and purchasing authorities). Thus, while you could select a hospital based on such issues as the visiting times on the ward, how much information you got, the quality of the food, the length of the waiting list, and how long you would have to stay in, you remained in the dark as to whether the surgeon in that hospital was actually any good at your operation. Not only had medical audit the potential to put power into the contracting process, it would also provide an incentive for doctors to improve their practices. However, the strength of the medical profession in keeping a closed shop on medical mistakes, the threat of litigation, and the profession's overriding belief in clinical freedom, have meant that instigating medical audit to improve consumer choice and bringing medical performance into the open are likely to be some way off.

Medical audit

Working Paper 6 (DoH, 1989b) defined medical audit as 'the systematic, critical analysis of the quality of medical care, including the procedures used for diagnosis and treatment, the use of resources, and the resulting outcome and quality of life for the patient', and stated that

> . . . medical audit must be *central* to any programme to enhance the overall quality of care given to patients in the NHS.

The language of the paper was designed to win over doctors to the concept of obligatory audit, by choosing not to highlight the hidden concept of accountability. It built on a slow movement already taking place in the medical profession towards audit. The emphasis was on the importance of medical audit as a medically-led initiative, and the Royal Colleges and the regional health authorities were given large sums of money for implementation. Audit was to be obligatory and to become part of consultant contracts.

Throughout the implementation plans, the Royal Colleges emphasised the principle that audit discussions were to remain confidential. The purpose of audit as seen by the Standing Committee on Postgraduate Medical Education (1989) was not managerial but educational, a view reinforced by the Royal College of Physicians (1989) who saw education as the 'most powerful product of audit'. Audit at this stage was still viewed therefore as a confidential tool for improving the standards of medical practice. Thus it met the requirements of performance review, but kept that process securely behind doctors' white coats.

The Department of Health (DoH) undoubtedly had a different understanding of the purpose of medical audit, stemming from a desire to restrain the soaring costs of the service, and a long and torrid history of attempts to make doctors accountable for their use of NHS resources, by involving them in the management of those resources. Such attempts included clinical budgeting, management budgeting and resource management (Packwood *et al*, 1990; Costain, 1989). All too often managers were of the belief that they were being asked to manage within limited resources with one hand tied behind their backs.

These two widely differing purposes reflect the long standing problem of the NHS defined by Klein (1982) as an attempt to 'combine the doctrine of public accountability with the doctrine of professional autonomy'. This dichotomy is reflected in the DoH's interpretation of audit as an integral part of the management process (Huntington, 1990). In the implementation of audit there have been initiatives to convince medical staff that audit presents opportunities for 'good medical practice, rather than . . . an attempt by management or medical colleagues to criticise practice in public or to threaten clinical freedom.' Bull (1990) argues that while general managers can expect to be given the general results of medical audit, and can request the auditing of specific areas, they must leave the doctors to examine the professional implications of the detailed results without 'the fear of premature intervention and penalty'. On the other hand, Maynard (1989) argues that the medical profession is not prepared radically to alter its education or service delivery, and therefore will not take on board the full implications of audit. Nixon (1990) reports in the *British Medical Journal* that the constraints on audit include doctors' attitudes, time, the cost of audit, and the problems of definition. Certainly time is of great importance, as doctors have not routinely included any peer review into their practice at consultant level. Thus, audit was supported and viewed as an add on to current medical duties, rather than a potential time saver and resource freer.

It is claimed that medical audit has improved communication between peers; improved working relationships between professional groups; improved collaboration between primary and secondary health care professionals; and improved the organisation of services (Frater, 1992). On this matter I would suggest the jury is still out. However, there is considerable commitment to medical audit from the NHS Management Executive, which has funded medical audit over and above baseline resources for four consecutive years.

The purpose of medical audit

As we have seen, different groups held different expectations of medical audit; this has created tensions in terms of the purpose of audit. These tensions and dilemmas were identified by Kerrison (1993) in the report

Medical audit – taking stock:

> Is it a process to monitor the provision of 'quality care' to satisfy those external to the organisation?

> Is it a professional educational process aimed at improving the practice of medicine by comparing individual practice with good professional standards?

> Is it a management process to contribute to the more effective use of resources within a hospital?

The report goes on to say that in attempting to satisfy or at least recognise more than one of these purposes, medical audit is unlikely to meet any one of them satisfactorily. To put it crudely, and to over-generalise, the conflicts that ensue arise from the different expectations of those who control the medical audit funding (the doctors), those who control the provision of services (the purchasers), those attempting to manage within the market (the providers), and those who believe in a more holistic approach to care (the nurses). Clinical audit must not fall into the same trap.

Nursing audit

Nurses make up the majority of the labour force of the NHS, and have the most patient contact, providing 24 hour direct patient care. Due to its size, nursing is also the most expensive service in terms of staffing costs. While doctors will be making costly decisions about patient care, nurses also have a part to play in the management of resources. This being the case, it would seem that nursing plays a significant part in the ability of a hospital to provide a value for money service.

While it is claimed by Salvage (1990) that nurses have the skills for audit, there has been little written about nursing audit. It differs from medical audit in one important aspect – it is used as a managerial function to evaluate the cost effectiveness of nursing, as well as for the professional development of practice and for education.

Brar (1989) identifies the objectives of nursing audit to be:

1. To justify the cost occurred on human and material resources.
2. To study the degree of quality patient care against defined criteria.
3. To take remedial actions towards cost effectiveness.

These have been expanded by Morison (1991) to include 'to foster in nurses a critical questioning approach to their activities and the needs of patients'. You can see the similarities in purpose to medical audit, but these are reconciled in an open dialogue between the professionals and the managers. It is common to link nursing audit to quality assurance programmes so that it is seen as an agent for improving quality (Elbeik and McGill, 1985). Thus the auditing of standards of nursing care is a central part of nursing audit (Girvin, 1990; Marker, 1988; Morison, 1991). 'Off the shelf' quality monitoring packages such as Monitor and QUALPACS (Sale, 1990) have been used as the first attempts to audit nursing in this country (Lorentzon, 1989), whereas prior work in the USA concentrated on chart or nursing records audit (Phaneuf, 1976). However, Jelinek *et al* (1974) soon discovered that nurses could learn to produce good documentation to influence the audit, and Hegyvary and Haussman (1976) argued that they could do this without improving patient care. While records audit in isolation is controversial, it can be useful as part of a more widely spread audit process. The philosophy of nursing is moving towards partnership with patients and, therefore, patients are commonly involved in the audit process (Allanach and Golden, 1988; Girvin, 1990). Distinctively, Orr and Bryant (1990) recommend that nursing audit should contain an action sheet to recognise what has been achieved, to develop ideas for improvement, and to make recommendations for action to be taken. An action sheet is already an integral part of the Doncaster Nursing Audit (1972). Thus nursing audit has moved on from records dependent audit, and incorporates the views of patients and the wider aspects of quality alongside clinical care.

Therapy audit

Therapists have found it difficult in some instances to access resources for audit. This reflects their general invisibility within the service, stemming from the fact that their numbers are small (unlike nursing) and they do not have a position by right at the Trust board table. However, therapy practices do lend themselves well to audit and, in fact, in many instances are much easier to audit than nursing interventions. Moreover, therapists have been developing measures for assessing the impact of their interventions on patient outcomes for some time, particularly in relation to functional assessment, with measures such as the Barthel Index (Mahoney and Barthel, 1965), and in the USA, through the development of a Uniform Data Set for Medical Rehabilitation (1990). Such scoring systems are a fundamental part of therapy evaluation.

The purpose of therapy interventions tends to have a clear definition and clear parameters and thus can be easily compartmentalised for audit purposes. Moreover, as therapy services are contracted for in terms of numbers of sessions, much as district nurses are contracted for in terms of numbers of contacts, there is a real need to demonstrate the effectiveness of those sessions in order to personalise the service and to define the expected outcomes. Therapists are finding that they are not always involved in determining their service contracts, thus doctors may be deciding the numbers of sessions required for a dietician or speech therapist, based on their expectations of how long it will take to treat the patient. The therapists then have to obtain a new referral if they need to see patients over and above the normal contracted service.

The small numbers of therapists makes the necessity for peer review involving therapists from potential competitor NHS Trusts crucial to performance improvement. The funding for this activity could be hard to define once audit finances are distributed to purchasers. The strength in therapy audit lies in its ability to obtain measures of outcomes relatively quickly; the fact that the small numbers mean that universal standards will be easier to introduce; and its willingness to collaborate with nurses to undertake cross-professional audit for patients requiring the services of both professions.

Clinical audit

Considerable interchangeable use was made of the terms clinical and medical as applied to audit. Clinical audit, however, is now interpreted as being multidisciplinary in nature. It was Trent Regional Health Authority (1990), in their plans for the implementation of medical audit, who identified the need to establish links between medical audit, clinical audit and quality assurance. This was to include extension of peer review to nurses, psychologists and paramedics. The recognition that audit had to encompass a multidisciplinary approach was stressed by the Royal College of Nursing (RCN) in its evidence on the White Paper to the Social Services Select Committee (Hancock, 1990). The RCN argument was that patients required the contribution of the whole professional team in their care and thus all members of that team should be subjected to audit. Howden (1990) argues that as a medical tool audit offers

> . . . limited scope in specialities where decision making and care are a matter of teamwork and it is methodologically impossible (as well as undesirable) to audit the contribution of one team member.

It is recognised by Shaw (1989) that, historically, doctors have included nurses and others in discussions about individual cases but that this needs to move away from subjective discussions towards objective and systematic review. He also argues that it is possible to audit a particular professional's work, so medical audit 'relates to practices initiated directly by doctors', and clinical audit covers the work of the team. The use of clinical audit complements the move into a purchaser/provider scenario (NHS Act 1990), where the health care needs of the population are assessed and appropriate services are provided (Mallett, 1991). Clinical audit requires a move away from the paternalistic attitude to the ward round or inviting nurses to the medical audit meeting. Clinical audit must recognise all participants in the process as partners and peers. It also requires some agreement between the professions on the priorities for clinical audit. Given the different interests and the differing views the professions have of the service they provide, this in itself will be a major challenge. Clinical audit must also find an agreed purpose, rather than bringing along the baggage of a single profession audit. It is a chance to learn the lessons of medical, nursing and therapy audit. Clinical audit is being instigated formally four years on from the inception of medical audit. In that time the NHS market has begun to throw up strengths in terms of its ability to improve the quality of services and weakness in the pattern of a two-tier service resulting from split purchasing. John Major, with his charters, has taken over the helm from Mrs Thatcher, though the policy thrust remains broadly similar. These events have contributed to a more qualified direction for audit as part of the rise of new public management.

New public management

Pollitt (1993) sums up the development of a second wave of reforms, started in the third Thatcher term, which has continued with the change in leadership of the government. These reforms known as 'new public management' are comprised of four main elements, namely: quasi-markets for services that could not be privatised; decentralisation; constant reference to the need to improve 'quality'; and the primacy of the wishes of the 'consumer'. The last two can be seen in the development of clinical audit from medical audit in that it is being heralded under the banner of quality and challenges audit to address the thorny issue of public accountability.

On 1 February 1993 Dr K Calman announced the first provision of funding for *clinical* audit. Both he and Mrs Moores, the Chief Nursing Officer for the DoH, and the Director of Nursing Services for the NHS ME, put audit firmly in the realms of quality. In both their statements they referred to audit as a mechanism for improving clinical care and quality of service. This is significant in that it presents a united front between the professions, at least at the centre, on the purpose of audit and enables clinical audit to break away from its previously protected status of internal professional peer review. The policy statement on clinical audit that followed later in the year continued this theme, and put consumerism firmly on the agenda as part of clinical audit development. The immediate challenge is to put clinical audit within quality as part of the contracting process, funded by purchasers in negotiation with providers. In order to do this, all parties require a common understanding of audit process, the relationship between audit and other central initiatives, the role of different professional groups, and the role of different organisations. The following chapters seek to address these issues.

References

Allenach E and Golden B (1988) Patients' expectations and values clarification: a service audit. *Nursing Administration Quarterly* **12** (3): 17–22.

Black N, Chapple J, Dalziel M, Spiby J (1989) Audit with kid gloves. *Health Services Journal*, 9 February: 176.

Brar A (1989) An evaluation of patient care. *The Nursing Journal of India* **80** (10): 189.

Bull A (1990) Doctors, managers and audit. *Health Services Management* **86** (6): 276.

Costain D (1989) Managing clinical activity. *Times Health Supplement*, September: 4.

Department of Health (1989a) *Working For Patients*. London: HMSO.

Department of Health (1989b) *Medical Audit – Working Paper No 6. Working for Patients*. London: HMSO.

Department of Health (1990) *Consultants, Contracts and Job Plans*. London: Health Circular HC (90) 16.

Doncaster Hospital Management Committee (1972) *Management Audit for the Nursing Services*, Doncaster Health Authority.

Elbeik M, McGill B (1985) Study reveals nursing audit can be a meaningful quality assurance tool. *Dimensions in Health Service* **62** (6): 31–32.

Ellis B, Rivett R, Dudley H (1990) Extending the use of clinical audit data. *British Medical Journal* **301**: 159–162.

Frater A (1992) Health outcomes: a challenge to the status quo. *Quality in Health Care* **1**: 87–88.

Girvin J (1990) Setting standards – uphill work. *Nursing Standard* **4** (44): 34–35.

Greenwood J, Wilson D (1989) *Public Administration in Britain Today*. London: Unwin Hyman.

Hancock C (1990) Can it work for patients? *Senior Nurse* **10** (7): 8–10.

Hegyvary S, Haussman R (1976) Monitoring nursing care quality. *Journal of Nursing Administration* **6** (9): 6–9.

Howden P, Chapman P, Waterfall A, Crown J (1990) A climate of trust. *The Health Services Journal* **100** (15): 402.

Huntington J (1990) In the pursuit of good quality. *The Health Services Journal* **100** (16): 521.

Jelinek D, Haussmann R, Hegyvary S (1974) *A Methodology for Monitoring Quality of Nursing Care*. US Department of Health, Education and Welfare, Bethesda, Maryland.

Kerrison S, Packwood T, Buxton M (1993) *Medical Audit Taking Stock*. London: King's Fund Centre.

Kitson A *et al* (1989) *A Framework for Quality*. London: Royal College of Nursing, RCN Publications.

Klein R (1982) Performance, evaluation and the NHS: a case study in conceptual perplexity and organisational complexity. *Public Administration* **60**, Winter 1982: 387.

Klein R (1989) *The Politics of the National Health Service*. London: Longman.

Lorentzon M (1989) *Nursing audit: a brief overview of some current developments*. Paper presented at North East Thames Regional Health Authority Seminar, November.

Mahoney R I and Barthel D W (1965) Functional evaluation: the Barthel Index. *Maryland State Medical Journal* **14**: 61–65.

Mallett J (1991) Shifting the focus of audit. *The Health Services Journal*, 28 February, 24–25.

Marker C (1988) The Marker Model for Nursing Standards: implications for nursing administration. *Nursing Administration Quarterly* **12** (2): 4–12.

Maynard A (1989) Audit: an Achilles' Heel. *The Health Services Journal*, 7 September, 1105.

Morison M (1991) The Stirling Model of Nursing Audit. *Professional Nurse*, April, 369.

National Association of Health Authorities (1990) Briefing, No 27.

NHS Management Executive (1991) *A Framework of Audit for Nursing Services*. London: HMSO.

Nixon S (1990) Defining essential hospital data. *British Medical Journal* **300**: 300–381.

Orr I and Bryant R (1990) Development of an audit system. *Senior Nurse* **10** (9): 14–15.

Packwood T, Buxton M, Keen J (1990) Resource management in the National Health Service: A first case history. *Policy and Politics* **18** (4): 245–255.

Packwood T, Keen J, Buxton M (1991) *Hospitals in Transition*. Milton Keynes: Open University Press.

Phaneuf M (1976) *The Nursing Audit*. New York: Appleton-Century-Crofts.

Pollitt C (1984) Blunt tools: performance measurement in policies for health care. *International Journal of Management Science* **12** (2): 131–140.

Pollitt C (1986) A poor performance. *New Society*, 3 October, 20–21.

Pollitt C (1993) *Managerialism and the Public Services*, 2nd Edn. Oxford: Blackwell Business.

Roberts H (1991) Measuring performance in the NHS. *Hospital Management International*: 94–104.

Royal College of Physicians (1989) *Medical Audit. A First Report. What, Why and How*. London: Royal College of Physicians.

Royal College of Surgeons of England (1989) *Guidelines to Clinical Audit in Surgical Practice*. London: Royal College of Surgeons.

Sale D (1990) *Quality Assurance*. London: Macmillan.

Salvage J (1990) Promoting good practice. *Nursing Standard*. **4** (4): 52–53.

Shaw C (1990) Criterion-based audit. *British Medical Journal* **300**: 649.

Shaw C and Costain D (1989) Guidelines for medical audit: seven principles. *British Medical Journal* **299**: 498.

Standing Committee on Postgraduate Medical Education (1989) *Medical Audit. The Educational Implications*. London: SCOPME.

Stevens G and Bennett J (1989) Clinical audit – occurrence screening for QA. *Health Services Management* **85** (4): 178–181.

Trent Regional Health Authority (1990) *Medical Audit Implementation Plans*.

Tugwell P and Mongonelli E (1986) The clinical audit cycle. *Australian Clinical Review*, June, 101–105.

Uniform Data System for Medical Rehabilitation and The Center for Functional Assessment Research (1990) *Guide for Use of the Uniform Data Set for Medical Rehabilitation*. Version 3.0. New York: State University of New York at Buffalo.

2

Getting Started on Audit

The process of audit

As described in Chapter 1, audit is a cycle of activity involving systematic review of practice, identification of problems, development of possible solutions, implementation of change, and then review again. When starting out on audit, many professionals assume that you begin with the measurement phase, or you start with setting standards. This in itself requires choice i.e. what standards do we start with? What do we measure? The common solution to these questions is for the professional groups to sit down and negotiate between them the topic to be audited. Immediately this causes problems. All too often, what one profession thinks is top of the priority list, another thinks is at the bottom. For example, the doctor may want to audit the efficiency of the endoscopy service, with the hidden agenda that he wants an extra nurse to recover patients. The nurse may want to audit patients' wound management with the hidden agenda for nursing to take a lead within the multidisciplinary team. The therapist may want to audit referrals, with the hidden agenda of improving GP letters and referral patterns. What one professional group thinks is easy to put straight, another thinks poses too many problems. For instance, the efficiency of the endoscopy service may be improved by many solutions other than increasing the nurse staffing numbers. In fact, that solution may be prohibited by resource constraints. What causes one individual grief is of little concern to another. One nurse may find it unacceptable that the ward is to become mixed sex. Another may view it as the only practical solution to bed management and thus believe it to be the best solution. Moreover, if audit topic selection is left to the professionals, it denies the patients a right to say what causes them the most concern and it excludes a managerial context which may be the make or break of the audit cycle. For instance, in the situation described above, the patient's main concern about the endoscopy service may be pain or lack of information. The patient in this situation becomes the passive contributor to feedback on an agenda set by health care professionals. We are rarely aware of our own inadequacies in putting ourselves in our patients' shoes.

All too often we think we know what patients feel without asking them. The managerial context in the case of the endoscopies may be that the activity is already too high in that area for the contract and the solution is to decrease endoscopy lists. So, is the answer to involve patients and managers in this group process for topic selection? If so, how do we make sure that the individuals attending are truly representative, or are empowered to say what they really think? I suggest that the historical pattern of audit topic selection by professionals is inadequate, and does not enable neutral territory for priority setting.

There is a need to prioritise audit topics, against criteria agreed by the whole team to be involved. CASPE Research and Brighton Health Care have developed criteria for the selection of audit projects. Any audit project in Brighton must meet the following criteria:

Does the project address a known quality issue?
Does the project address an important area of practice?
Is there an achievable quality improvement?
Does the project address an area of clinical certainty and consensus?
Will the project test, use or set explicit standards?
Does the project have clinical support?
Does the project involve self-audit?
Is the project multidisciplinary? (Walshe and Tomlin, 1993)

The key criterion for audit should be that if you can't change it, don't audit it. Any approach to audit must include an understanding of the planning and process of change. Change is the key link in the audit cycle. It is often easy to measure or set standards but it is much harder to change clinical and managerial practices in the light of the measurement findings. Broome (1990) describes the open systems theory which proposes that no change can be implemented without consideration of the wider environment which places demands on the system and to which it must respond. Thus, if attempting to change clinical practice in relation to wound care, consideration must be taken of the interests of the patients, managers and health care professionals. An audit of wound care may call for more patient self care and information, fewer staff undertaking the dressings, better equipment or dressings, more appropriate prescription, a handover of responsibility from one professional group to another and so on. Change in any one area can be advanced or hindered by one of the aforementioned groups.

Moreover, outcomes of care cannot be considered in isolation from the human systems in which they take place. They are dependent on those systems, a factor of the processes put in place and cannot be abstracted from those processes. Therefore, in order to audit it is essential to have an understanding of the planning and process of change as well as an understanding of the climate in which creative solutions to problems can be reached. In order to use audit to evaluate the nursing and therapy contribution to the service, there must be the opportunities in the organisation for nurses and therapists to develop their practices and for the management of these practices to reach their real potential. Without the commitment to planned change, audit becomes yet another punitive stick with which to beat the professional, rather than an opportunity to develop and improve services. All too often, support for audit is only prevalent in measuring and reviewing current practice and nurses and therapists are expected to undertake change without the necessary facilitation and leadership. This chapter starts by exploring current change theories, relating them to audit, and suggests a model and framework for change. Once a model is adopted, the rest of the difficulties in relation to audit fall into place. The key to getting started on audit is to begin at what would seem to be the end of the first trip round the cycle – the implementation of change.

Change theories

Bennis dominates the field of theory related to change. Bennis *et al* (1976) describe three strategies for change as rational–empirical, power–coercive, and normative–re-educative. Rational–empirical assumes that people are rational and self-interested, and will view change in a positive way as long as they perceive some personal benefits. Power–coercive relies on the power to direct others requiring only their compliance. Usually the power is that of authority, and is described as the 'top down' approach (Wright, 1989). Lastly normative–re-educative requires participation in change, based on a new understanding of current practices, and a commitment to formulating new approaches. The strategy requires direction but involves delegation of responsibility. This latter approach to change fits comfortably with the cycle of audit as it supports reviewing practices, by the nursing team and a problem solving approach to development.

Chin (Bennis *et al*, 1976) developed three analytical models of change: the system model, the developmental model, and the model for changing. The system model emphasises stability and proposes that change comes about as a result of stress or tension in a system. Thus the purpose of change in this model is to reaffirm stability. The developmental model accepts that change is a natural part of life and as such is never ending. The last model uses both previous approaches, focusing on the forces producing change. It is important that, when undertaking audit, nurses understand the reasons for it and the forces on their environment that will impact their decision making when planning change.

Change is not easy – like the grieving process, there are stages that all staff undergo which must be recognised and supported in order for that change to be successful. Hersey and Blanchard (1977) describe four levels of change, which become increasingly difficult to achieve. These are knowledge change, attitudinal change, behavioural change and, lastly, group or organisational performance change. Historically, audit has sought to achieve knowledge change, with the assumption that as an educational process, change in behaviour would then follow. However, this achieves only the easiest of the levels of change and, as we are beginning to find out, makes little impact on the service. The frustration, particularly with medical audit, is that the return on investment looks poor. The reality is that to improve services we need to recognise the difficulties and challenges in changing attitudes, behaviour and, lastly, performance. These take a considerable time, particularly if we are talking about changing whole group performance. For instance, discharge audits may result in the need to change record keeping to improve the planning process, record storage, medical practice in relation to GP letters, nurse to nurse communication, the post room to ensure that communication reaches to right address and so on.

The change process is described as a cycle by Rogers (1962) with five phases: awareness, interest, evaluation, trial and adoption. Kelly and Corner (1979) also describe a cycle, but an emotional cycle. This involves the phases of uninformed optimism, informed pessimism, hopeful realism, informed optimism and rewarding completion. This is all too obvious in the audit cycle. At the outset, the participants are optimistic about how they will fare in the process. When they get the audit results, they find they are not doing as well as they thought. Having come to terms with these facts, they then begin to plan how to improve their care in the light of their current situation. They tackle the problem head on and, having achieved their goals, at the end of the cycle they have managed to reach the standard they aspired to. Three other phases of change, those of unfreezing, moving and refreezing (Lewin, 1951), involve developing an awareness of the need for change, working towards change and, finally, the integration of the change and its subsequent stabilisation. In relation to audit this is vital. The measurement phase will create a need for change, but only if the participants are willing to recognise that need. Once they are convinced, they then need to plan the change process, work on it and ensure it becomes standard day by day practice.

Planned change

We have seen that the change process is vital to the success of the audit cycle. However, change in itself should be planned and systematically implemented otherwise there is the risk of failure and disillusionment with the audit process. Change in audit is planned as a result of the review of current practice against agreed standards. Bennis *et al* (1976) describe planned change as 'conscious, deliberate, and a collaborative effort to improve the operations of a human system'. When planning change, Vaughan (1989) suggests that there are two areas for consideration, the individuals concerned and the organisation. This is supported by Beyers (1984) who believes that the first step in approaching change is to assess where nursing fits into the organisation. Bailey and Claus (1975) compare change to problem solving, and advocate a systems approach. Broome (1990) describes the open systems theory which proposes that no change in a system can be implemented without consideration of the wider environment which places demands on the system, and to which it must respond. Thus, if attempting to change practice on a ward, consideration must be given to the interests of the patients, organisation and other professional groups. Neglecting these factors jeopardises the ability to make lasting change that becomes parts of everyday work patterns. Bennis (1976) asserts that planned change entails 'mutual goal setting, an equal power ratio (eventually), and deliberateness on both sides'. In other words, if change is going to take place in a multidisciplinary team, all members of that team should be viewed as equals in achieving that change. It should not be the assertion of the will of one professional group over another. This will only mean that the underdog will subvert the change at any opportunity. The strategy for change should ensure that there is ownership of the change by the participants and that the change appeals to the participants' values as well as to their rational being. Thus, all those expected to implement the change should be involved from the outset. Kelly and Corner (1979) argue that all resistance to change stems from fear, thus participation and understanding reduce resistance. This is particularly so in audit. Professionals view audit with trepidation, as they are afraid it will expose personal and professional inadequacies. They also fear punitive action if the audit shows less than satisfactory results. It is, therefore, important to ensure all staff involved in the service to be audited are: familiar with, or contribute to the design of, the measurement tools to be used; that all staff contribute to the standard setting process, either directly or through consultation; that all staff understand the purpose and process of the audit. This preparation is time consuming but worthwhile. All too often we hear of enthusiastic staff unable to generate enthusiasm for the audit in others. All too often we hear of staff non-participation in gathering audit data. This is due to poor preparation and lack of motivation to take part.

Other factors that contribute to successful change are described as: open exchange of information, opinion and feelings (Mauksch and Miller, 1981); the lower the risk the more likely it is to succeed (Rogers and Shoemaker, 1971); ownership and adoption of the values of the change (Bennis, 1976; Wright, 1989); focusing on one step at a time (Hickman et al, 1984); using the critical mass (the least number to make the change happen) (Broome,

1990); and nurturing the participants (Lancaster and Lancaster, 1982). All change takes time if it is to be successful beyond the involvement of its champion. Recognising that fact and planning for it makes the process more satisfactory and does not raise expectations prematurely.

The change agent

In order to achieve planned change the strategy adopted requires leadership in the form of a change agent (Bennis, 1976). A change agent is the person whose specific role is to assist in the change effort (Pearson, 1895). This person is crucial to the success of the change, supporting participants during the risky phases of change, generating ideas, reducing resistance, and evaluating the change (Broskawski, 1975). The change agent's role is described by Lancaster and Lancaster (1982) as: diagnosis of the problems; assessment of the participants and his own motivation and capacity; selection of objectives and ways to achieve these; determination of his own role; maintenance of change; and, finally, withdrawal. It is proposed by Sheehan (1990) that change agents serve three functions. Firstly they prepare the way for change, then they facilitate its implementation and, lastly, they repair the 'breakdowns'. All too often audit takes place without change agents, or with ineffective change agents. For instance, audit officers are sometimes seen as responsible for audit but they have neither the training in change management, nor the credibility or authority with the whole multidisciplinary team. In nursing there has been a dramatic increase in the number of practice development nurses employed to take responsibility for changing nursing practice. This is not a managerial position, rather the development nurse works as a support nurse to the Trust nurse (thus occupying a senior position within the Trust), while collaborating with clinical nurses in exploring new ways of working, or implementing research findings. These nurses work at all levels of the organisation, with credibility as practitioners and change agents.

These descriptions of the role of the change agent seem to infer the acceptance of Chin's previously described 'model for changing' which requires the change agent to stimulate change. It is argued that the characteristics of the change agent should include creativity or the generation of new ideas, founded on a basis of familiarity with the issues (Henry and Walker, 1991). In order to create excellence Hickman et al (1984) propose that six skills are required. These are 'creative insight, sensitivity, vision, versatility, focus, and patience'. They also describe five steps in implementing change, which are: defining the change; determining who and/or what need to change; determining the resources required; planning the pathway; beginning to implement the change incorporating on-going monitoring and review. These skills are critically lacking in nursing practice. Any attempt to plan change will require the training of the change agents to provide them with the key abilities for leading practice. Without change agents, audit is likely to fail and their key skill must lie in the familiarity with the issues. The issues as they relate to audit will be managerial, professional, organisational and environmental. Thus the change agent must be able to span the organisation, to get an understanding of the context in which change must take place.

Climate for change

Determining the who, what and how for the change phase of the audit cycle requires problem solving (Bailey and Claus, 1975). This requires an organisational climate in which the creative solutions to problems can be generated. The measurement phase can thus be used as a 'springboard to innovation' (Henry and Walker, 1991). Such a climate is one where groups are allowed some degree of independence from high level interference. It requires open communication systems, network-forming arrangements and decentralisation of resources (Moss Kanter, 1985). Other elements are participation and freedom of expression (Bower, 1965), flexibility and sensitivity (Handy, 1985). This climate is far from apparent in many organisations but can be developed with the help of the change agent. It requires decentralised decision making and practitioners/clinicians having control over their own practice. In order to create this climate for change in clinical audit, the team undergoing audit must be cohesive. In many instances, preparatory team building exercises will lay the bedrock for audit to incorporate successful change.

A model for change

In order to implement the audit process, a strategy for change has to be determined which incorporates a theoretical model. Once the strategy is agreed, the audit methodology for data collection can be designed to meet the strategy's requirements. The 'model for changing' identifies the need to consider the forces that affect change. These forces are the interests of the patients, the organisation, and the professions (Figure 2.1). Thus, when designing methodology, it is important to gather information on these interests as they relate to the area being audited. They are complex, and often conflicting. Put simply, the organisation's interests relate to: the necessity to provide value for money in order to attract contracts for services; the patients' interests relate to being empowered through information; the doctors' interests relate to treating the patients as quickly and effectively as possible in a medical model, and to maintaining their status;

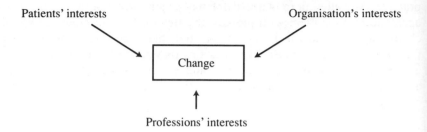

Figure 2.1 The forces that affect change

the nurses' interests are to demonstrate the importance of their contribution to the quality of patient care and to develop a therapeutic holistic model of care; and the therapists' interests are to retain a professional model for therapy services incorporating autonomy in the treatment process.

In designing an audit of the care of patients who have had a stroke, clinical care will only be one factor. It is important when gathering information about the clinical care also to gather information in relation to:

a) The organisation's expectations (i.e. the contracted length of stay, where it is expected care will take place, the quality standards in the contract).
b) The staff's concerns (possibly the lack of privacy for care, lack of equipment, the fact that therapy services are only available during weekdays, the different expectations of the professions in relation to goal setting).
c) The patient's or carer's concerns (possibly lack of dignity, loss of familiar routine, pain, lack of understanding or information on progress or planned goals).

This information will help prioritise those areas that need changing and can be changed. It provides the context to clinical care and often provides the reasons why clinical care is not as good as expected. All too often it is not the prescription of care that is at fault or the intentions of the staff, rather, it is a mis-match between the expectations of the organisation, staff and patient/carer. This contextual information can be gathered in a variety of ways. In this instance, if we are considering the care of a patient who has had a stroke in a hospital setting, then the information on staff expectations may be common to all the client groups being cared for in that setting. This information can be used to consider the need for change not just for patients who have had a stroke but for all patients in that ward. The methodology for collecting data for each of these expectations/concerns could be as follows:

a) Organisation's expectations. Gather data against the contract standards (quality, productivity). Interview senior managers on their expectations for next year's contracts for this service – there is little point making the effort to develop a service that is to diminish or become redundant. There again, the audit may point the service in a new direction that would attract contracts.

b) Staff expectations. Find out what the staff think of the service now through an anonymous questionnaire. How do the staff want to progress care over the next year? Are they planning to introduce a new way of working (e.g. Primary Nursing)? This will affect the audit's recommendations for change.

c) Patients'/carers' concerns. Questionnaires given out while the patient is still in hospital will not give an accurate picture of the patient's concerns. Rather it will pick up positive messages on the staff attitude and you will think all is well. This is not helped by the fact that staff tend to design questionnaires that reflect their own concerns, rather than allowing patients to express theirs (e.g. questionnaires that ask patients to tick boxes about the information they were given and the temperature of the food, but exclude questions on pain or whether they understood the information). A more accurate response will be elicited if patients and/or carers are interviewed after discharge from the hospital when they have had time to reflect on their experience and put it into the context of their real lives. Interviews that are open and allow patients to set the agenda are the most likely to achieve the desired result. It must be noted, however, that in the current climate, patients are being bombarded with questions, so make sure that they have not already been interviewed, find out what interviews have already taken place in the hospital, and put your interview schedule through the local ethics committee.

The central themes arising from the literature are that audit is a cycle of activity which should enable the development of practices that provide value for money. The methodology for data collection should produce information to enable the change strategy to incorporate the interests of the organisation, the doctors and the patients, as well as of the nursing and/or therapy team to be audited (Open Systems Approach). The strategy should also incorporate a change agent who undertakes to manage the audit cycle. The normative–re-educative change process seems to facilitate successful change, and would best fit the concept of developing practice. The organisation's commitment to supporting effective nursing and therapy audit will need to commence with the development of change agent posts and with effective educational programmes for the post holders to develop the key skills required to lead change.

Audit is the development arm of research and development work. It is about the development of services in the light of research findings, and thus the links to research are tangible and important in planning audit programmes.

Research and audit

Audit has many similarities with research, but also many important differences. Unlike research, audit does not necessarily extend the knowledge base of medicine but by critically analysing medical practices audit aims to improve the quality of care. (*Making Medical Audit Effective*, 1992)

While audit may use research methodology (i.e. questionnaires, interview techniques) as part of the measurement phase of the cycle, audit itself is not research. Rather, it is the evaluation of the application of research findings in practice. In order to evaluate this application, audit should be comparing practice with research-based standards. In order to produce research-based standards, those setting the standards should have the ability to appraise published research critically, or rely on nationally recognised research programmes. Moreover, the provider unit's research programmes should recognise the importance of replicated research, and audit itself may identify areas that require further research and which should be fed back into the research agenda (Figure 2.2).

Mostly, audit is compared to biomedical research as this is the type of study predominantly undertaken by doctors and which in health care attracts the bulk of research funding. In making comparators between audit and biomedical research (i.e. clinical trials approach) we can see the differences (Figure 2.3).

This takes a positivist approach to research in that it is dependent on the concepts of observable, testable phenomena which achieve a positive stage

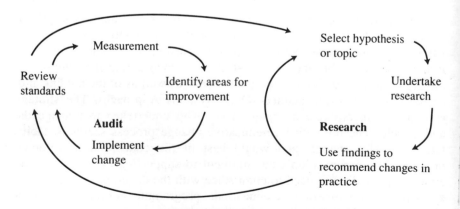

Figure 2.2 The relationship between audit and research

Audit	Research
Is not randomised	Is randomised
Compares actual performance against standards	Identifies the best approach, and thus sets the standards
Conducted by those providing the service	Not necessarily conducted by those providing the service
Usually led by service providers	Usually initiated by researchers
Does not involve instigation of new treatments but evaluates current treatments	Involves comparitors between new treatments and placebos
Involves review of records by those entitled to access them	Requires access by those not normally entitled to access
Does not necessarily have to be endorsed by the ethics committee, unless patients are to be personally involved (e.g. through interviews)	Must be endorsed by the ethics committee
Results not usually transferable to other settings	Results are generalisable to other settings
Uses tested hypothesis to develop standard Compares performance against standard	Determines a testable hypothesis grounded in empirical data Presents clear conclusions

Figure 2.3 The differences between audit and research

of development. However, this approach to research is not the only one. Social science research allows social interaction and has a lower level of precision and certainty than natural sciences (Weber, 1949). Rather than assume a hypothesis, in social science research it is possible to search the literature for generalisations and use them to build up a theoretical model. It is also acceptable to use both quantitative and qualitative methods. One such method which has similarities to some types of audit (particularly organisational audit) is the case study. This allows a holistic view of the current situation arising from the perspective of all parties involved (Yin, 1984). As such it is viewed as an inquiry (Denzin, 1978). It can be designed around the participants and involves both quantitative and qualitative methods. Case studies are concerned with the interaction of factors and events over a period of time and often have several embedded units of analysis. The case study approach can elicit from the literature the factors affecting the organisation's or individual profession's ability to change and can then structure methodology around the vital forces in a change model.

This fits in well with audit, if it is viewed essentially as an agent for change or improvement. It is possible to suggest that by using a case method approach to audit, it is possible to prioritise those areas that require detailed clinical audit. On a more practical note, in patient-focused audit, any patient questionnaires and interviews should go through the local ethics committee. Just because the enquiry is for audit, it doesn't make it immune from the ethical process. In determining priorities for areas requiring audit, it is vital that the national research and development strategy and the strategy for nursing research are considered. These will set a future agenda for audit by providing the research base to standards. Audit will be vital to observe the application of research undertaken as part of this strategy.

Consumer involvement in audit

> It is becoming increasingly accepted that the patient's perspective is critical in assessing the effectiveness of health care, and experience in polling patients on different aspects of their health, quality of life, or satisfaction with treatment is growing. (Bardsley and Coles, 1992)

Audit or, more precisely, medical audit has not generally considered patients' views. However, patients' views are now being sought about the quality of the service provided by purchasers, providers and professionals. Patients' perceptions of care are seen to be less controversial, provide a ready source of data, and identify issues that are easy to understand; health care professionals can respond to this information (Steven, 1991).

Anderson (1989) says:

> The difference between the provider of health services and the patient resembles that between the hen and the pig in the preparation of eggs and bacon. The hen is involved but the pig is committed.

The Patient's Charter is part of the rise of the 'new public management' commitment to consumerism. There is a tendency for off the shelf questionnaires of patient satisfaction to identify only the shop face of the service or superficial issues, rather than the care delivered. For example, questionnaires usually ask about the catering, signposting, parking and named nurses. While these are important they are not necessarily the patient's prime concern. Patient satisfaction is more likely to relate to whether the treatment and care solved their problems, relieved their symptoms or cured their illnesses. Thompson (1983) found that high levels of overall satisfaction were normally correlated with satisfaction with the *content* of care, whereas high levels of dissatisfaction were normally related to the *context* of care. It is thus easy to concentrate on the contextual issues, as these tend to claim false importance, rather than the content issues that are likely to have far reaching effects in terms of the patient's lifestyle. Eliciting patients' views on the content of their care requires a more open style of questioning and relates to their often low expectations of the service. It requires patients to explore what they have a right to expect, rather than assuming that all health service professionals do a good job. This is a more active view of consumerism as patient driven. Patient satisfaction could be seen as an indicator of service outcome.

A Total Quality Management system is centrally concerned with user preferences and published standards. The inclusion of patients/clients personally in the review process has been avoided by doctors. However, Richardson *et al* (1990) urge that the patient's perspective be included in audit to provide a consumer focus. Fitzpatrick (1991) suggests that patient satisfaction is an important outcome measure and provides valuable information on which to review practice and management. Thus, patients should be involved in the audit process as part of the assessment of outcomes. Patients could also be involved in setting priorities for audit. There are moves to involve them even more closely in the monitoring of audit and in assessing the results. The inclusion of a patients' representative on the NHS Management Executive Clinical Outcomes Group gives clear signals to the service about patient involvement.

Where to start

The Open Systems Approach requires us to find out the concerns and interests of all those involved in the clinical area and the factors that cause stess or tension in the system. In the Open Systems Model a ward might have a range of tensions (Figure 2.4).

Some of the tensions that each of these creates may be as follows

The organisation's plans   There may be plans to close the ward for redecorating; to turn it from a surgical ward into a medical ward; to put all the minor surgery into day cases; to upgrade the ward; to reduce staffing costs; to increase throughput and bed occupancy.

Staff morale   The staff's morale will enhance or diminish their performance. Thus their ability to do the job bears a direct relationship to their satisfaction with the job.

Professional aspirations   The nurses may want to move towards a decentralised system for caseload management (e.g. primary nursing); the doctors may want more control over the patient's experience and want the nurses to take on junior doctors' work to help reduce their hours; the therapists may want to provide an open referral system.

Patients' expectations and concerns   The patients' experiences and concerns may not be those of the staff. They may feel disempowered, alone,

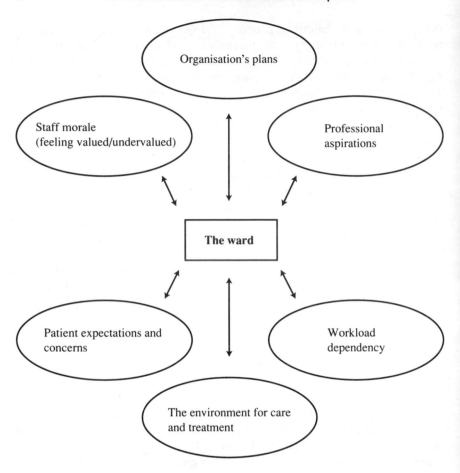

Figure 2.4 The ward

and without adequate information. They may be disappointed with the results of their stay; but may be happy to put up with things that the staff find unacceptable; they may want to stay in longer, or go home earlier. They are interested in the effectiveness of their treatment and whether it has improved things in their eyes. They may have different expectations of the outcomes of the ward stay.

Workload   The ability of the staff to improve their practice may be limited by the relationship between the demands of the patients and the supply of appropriate staff. It is also dependent on the numbers of actual admissions and discharges, and the severity of the patient's condition on arrival.

The environment   The inability to care is inextricably linked with the equipment availability (i.e. drip counters, lifting aids, treatment equipment) and the layout of the ward (including numbers and location of toilets)

Once all these concerns are elicited, it is possible to determine an agenda for change that seeks common solutions to problems and which prioritises areas that require detailed standards, with regular auditing.

Thus, we are setting a baseline of 'where are we at now?' against which we can compare ourselves annually, making a universal audit cycle for the clinical area. From this baseline, we are able to implement change to improve common or crucial problems. We can also set standards that

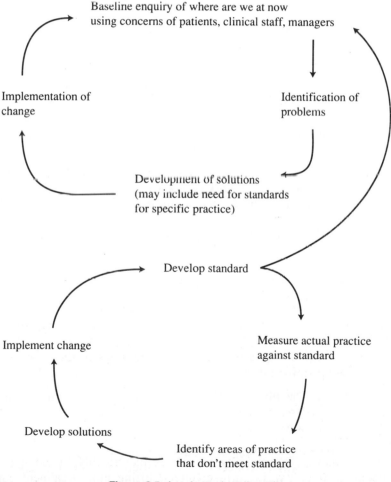

Figure 2.5 A universal audit cycle

require review on a more frequent basis (i.e. audit cycles within the audit cycle) but which can also be built into our baseline review the next year (Figure 2.5).

The baseline enquiry could thus consist of:

Organisational interview – ask the managers what their plans are for the ward, and undertake a SWOT analysis of these. Or, use your business plan to identify the major areas of change that the ward will have to manage.

Staff questionnaire – this could comprise: a structured morale and motivation section; a section that asks the respondent to list the 10 most satisfying things and the 10 most dissatisfying things (in order of priority) about working in the clinical area; a section that asks for open comment on the structured section. (See Appendix 1 – adapted from Humphries and Turner 1989.)

Professional interview – ask the leaders of each of the professions in your ward to identify where they think the service is going and their aspirations for the profession.

Patient interview – this could be administered after the patients' discharge from the service, when their difficulties or successes are most likely to be coming to the fore, and when they feel there is some distance between their current situation and the service they are being asked to comment on. An interview schedule might look like Appendix 2.

Workload – your manager or yourself will have details of your ward or service's throughput and staff workload. This should be available through resource management or the patient administration system. If not, then undertake a simple analysis of workload, using an off the shelf package. You should also incorporate some measure of clinical performance against his workload.

Clinical indicators – most clinical areas collect details of pressure sore prevalence, hospital acquired infections (such as wound and chest infections) and post-operative DVT rate. This information on morbidity is usually collected by the doctors if not by the nurses and therapists. It is important to pick clinical indicators that are reliant on the whole team's input. Chest infections are a reflection of the abilities of the anaesthetist, the physiotherapist, the junior doctor and the nurse.

The environment – health and safety audits of the environment should be available to you. Also the estates department may have access to a package that assesses your ward environment.

Given that we are not setting any boundaries on eliciting these opinions, it is vital to find a way of collecting information in a way that gives the respondent maximum flexibility while allowing data analysis. Thus, it is

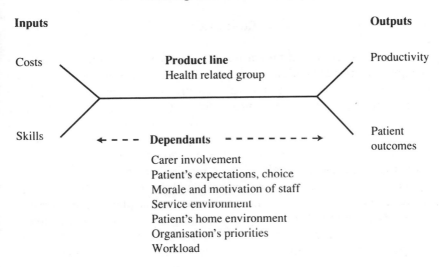

Figure 2.6 The value for money equation

probably better where possible to use scheduled interviews with open questioning rather than questionnaires. If it is seen as necessary to ensure that the respondent is not inhibited, it may be useful to get external help in administering the interviews, or revert to a questionnaire that does not constrain the response but allows for comments.

The value for money equation (Figure 2.6) demonstrates that if you put in the same skills and resources to a particular clinical process of care, you may not get the same outputs – i.e. productivity and patient outcomes (patient satisfaction and clinical outcomes). This is due to the fact that the process of care may not reflect the research in that area; the patient may not have the same expectations of that care process (he may not want his leg ulcer healed); the carer input is different in each patient; the environment of care affects the ability to achieve the required outcomes (continence on an elderly people's ward is a function of the amount of toilets within walking distance); morale and motivation of the staff plays an important factor in the quality of their work (Handy, 1985). All of these have the ability to hinder or enhance the care process and the outcomes of care. Any audit of outcome must therefore consider the inputs to care, process of care, and those factors that enable or hinder the staff. (The equation is explored further in Chapter 4.) This forms the basis for organisational audit and for setting more detailed audit priorities. In identifying priorities the negotiators need to have a view on the overall performance of the system, and those areas in which it is possible to affect change.

Conclusion

The history of clinical audit identifies the discrepancies in opinion about its managerial and/or educational function. The process of audit, encompassing a cycle of activity which involves measurement and change, enables the advancement of practice to improve the quality of care. The literature identifies some work in the application of audit to nursing but this has tended to focus on the measurement phase of the cycle. In order to evaluate and improve the professional's contribution to care, an understanding of the change phase of the audit cycle is required. In developing audit, the context in which treatment and care is undertaken must be taken into consideration. Moreover, patients' concerns should play a central part in prioritising audit topics. One way of capturing these factors while creating a planned approach to change is to develop a baseline review audit for the care area, or care team, that is administered regularly (e.g. annually). This should provide data on the context. From this, specific audit topics for detailed review can be selected and incorporated as part of an ongoing monitoring process into the baseline review the following year. This approach allows planned developments and achievements. It creates a positive climate for audit and contributes to team working. It addresses the difficulties in undertaking change and provides a realistic audit framework.

References

Anderson J (1989) Patient power in mental health. *British Medical Journal*, Dec 16: 1477–8.

Bailey J T and Claus K E (1975) *Decision Making in Nursing.* St Louis: CV Mosby Co.

Bardsley M and Coles J (1992) Practical experiences in auditing patient outcomes. *Quality in Health Care* 1 (2): 124–130.

Bennis W, Benne K, and Chin R (1976) *The Planning of Change*, 3rd Edn. London: Holt, Reinhart & Winston Inc.

Beyers M (1984) Getting on top of organisational change. *The Journal of Nursing Administration*, October 14 (12): 32–39.

Bower M (1965) Nurturing innovation in an organisation. In G A Steiner (Ed), *The Creative Organisation*, Chicago: Chicago University Press.

Broome A (1990) *Managing Change.* London: Macmillan.

Browskawski A, Mermis W J, and Khajavi F (1975) Managing the dynamics of change and stability. In Jones J E and Pfeiffer J W *The 1975 Annual Handbook for Group Facilitators.* California: University Associates Inc.

Fitzpatrick R (1991) Surveys of patient satisfaction. *British Medical Journal* 302: 887–889.

Handy C (1985) *Understanding Organisations*, 3rd Edn. London: Penguin Business.

Henry J and Walker D (1991) *Managing Innovation*. London: The Open University /Sage Publications.

Hersey P and Blanchard K H (1977) *Management of Organisational Behavior*. New Jersey: Prentice Hall.

Hickman C and Silva M (1984) *Creating Excellence*. London: George Allen & Unwin.

Humphries G and Turner A (1989) Job satisfaction and attitudes of nursing staff on a unit for the elderly infirm, with change of location. *Journal of Advanced Nursing* **14**: 298–307.

Joint Centre for Education in Medicine (1992) *Making Medical Audit Effective*. London: Joint Centre for Education in Medicine.

Kelly D and Corner D R (1979) The emotional cycle of change. In Jones J E and Pfeiffer J W *The 1975 Annual Handbook for Group Facilitators*. California: University Associates Inc.

Lancaster J and Lancaster W (1982) *The Nurse as Change Agent*. St Louis: CV Mosby Co.

Lewin K (1951) *Field Theory in Social Science* New York: Harper & Row Publications.

Marriner-Tomey A (1988) *A Guide to Nursing Management*, 3rd Edn. St Louis: CV Mosby Co.

Mauksch I and Miller M (1981) *Implementing Change in Nursing*. St Louis: CV Mosby Co.

Moss Kanter E (1985) *The Change Masters*. London: Unwin Paperbacks.

Pearson A (1985) Nurses as change agents and a strategy for change. *Nursing Practice* **2**: 80–84.

Richardson J, Stott R, and Rentoul R (1990) Gaining perspective. *The Health Services Journal*, 22 March: 435.

Rogers E (1962) *Diffusion of Innovations*. New York: The Free Press of Glencoe.

Rogers E and Shoemaker F (1971) *Communication of Innovations: a cross cultural approach*. New York: The Free Press of Glencoe.

Romano C (1990) Innovation. *Computers in Nursing*, May/June: 99–103.

Sheehan J (1990) Investigating change in a nursing context. *Journal of Advanced Nursing* **15**: 819–824.

Steven I (1991) A patient satisfaction questionnaire as a teaching and comparative audit tool. *Quality Assurance in Health Care* **3**: (1) 41–49.

Stevenson D (1990) The energy crisis of change. *Nursing Practice* **2**: 15–17.

Thompson A (1983) *The Measurement of Patients' Perception of the Quality of Hospital Care*. Unpublished doctoral thesis, University of Manchester.

Tugwell P and Mongonelli E (1986) The clinical audit cycle. *Australian Clinical Review* June: 101–105.

Vaughan B and Pillmoor M (1989) *Managing Nursing Work*. London: Scutari Press.

Walshe K and Tomlin D (1993) Raincheck: selecting, planning, implementing and evaluating audit projects. *Health Services Journal* **103** (5350): 28–29.

Weber M (1949) *Methodology of the Social Sciences*. New York: Free Press.

West M and Farr J (1990) *Innovation and Creativity at Work*. Chichester: John Wiley & Sons.

Wright S (1985) Change in nursing: the application of change theory to practice. *Nursing Practice* **2**: 85–91.

Wright S (1989) *Changing Nursing Practice*. London: Edward Arnold.

3

Audit Methodologies

Audit had its origins in the world of finance with the review of accounts undertaken by an external expert assessor. The concept of data review by experts has also been used in medicine for some time.

In the UK prior to the NHS reforms of 1989, medical audit was restricted to scrutiny of individual case notes by an 'expert' panel when complaints of negligent care could not be resolved at local level. The panel (known as 'three wise men' in the USA) were senior consultants who could comment authoritatively on the case under scrutiny.

Nursing took the lead on quality measurement in the 1980s with the introduction of American audit packages (Phaneuf, 1976) or anglicised versions, such as *Monitor* (Goldstone *et al*, 1983). Phaneuf's Audit was a retrospective review of nursing records, whereas *Monitor* incorporated observation of nurses at work and therefore also highlighted the processes of care delivery.

Many of the earlier audit approaches were derived from Donabedian's (1986) model of structure, process and outcome measurement. Organisational audit, in keeping with the American model of Accreditation of Services, involves the setting of organisational standards in consultation with an expert group.

Organisational audit

The standards written for organisational audit will reflect the mission statement and goals of the organisation. They express succinctly the intentions of the organisation in relation to the service it is attempting to provide. For example:

All personnel shall be prepared, through appropriate education and training programmes, for their responsibilities in the provision of a quality service.

The clinical directorates ensure that the collaborative care planning is used to design and provide appropriate care to meet the individual needs of patients/clients.

All clients will be treated with confidentially, courtesy and dignity.

Each of these statements reflects a promise by the organisation to provide a predetermined level of service. The core standards can be further refined at departmental level with criteria specific to each area.

Organisational audit differs from nursing/therapy audit in that the standards reflect core elements of the overall service, often relating to structure or process elements, whereas nursing/therapy audit has focused on clinical standards, with emphasis on outcomes and/or processes of care. Organisational audit provides a framework for comprehensive review of services and ensures consistency of approach and interpretation for quality across the organisation. The organisation's standards can be used in contracts between purchaser and provider to reflect the commitment to quality assurance.

Organisational audit differs from accreditation in that it is a local agreement reached between individual purchasers and provider units. However, the principles could be used to develop national organisational standards to facilitate accreditation.

The USA Joint Commission of Health Care Organisations is a well-established body which encourages hospitals to audit their practice against pre-set standards and criteria. This body has the authority to withdraw accreditation if standards are not at the accepted level, thus virtually putting the organisation out of business. The King's Fund approach to accreditation has involved developing an English version, which takes the best of the American and Australian systems without the same degree of punitive control. Organisations audited by the King's Fund pay for the privilege but are given opportunity to make up their shortfall in a given time frame following audit visits.

The advantages of organisational audit to an internal market must be the clear specification of intent, which provides tangible evidence against which performance, cost effectiveness and quality can be measured. The King's Fund Organisational Audit Project (1990) has led the field with many pilot projects in the UK. With the NHS Reforms (DoH, 1989) the demand for formal systems to measure quality and the emphasis on 'health care gains' as depicted in *Health of the Nation* (DoH, 1992) has led to a flurry of interest in establishing criteria for good care by provider units with which to impress and capture contracts from purchasing authorities.

The shift to patient focused clinical audit has resulted in the development of methods which focus on outcomes of care, and which may be used as standards or behavioural health status indicators. Behavioural health status indicators are those which convey a change in the functional ability of the client/patient, i.e. tangible change in their performance as a result of intervention/treatment. This set of indicators is therefore client focused and is a measure of outcomes.

Most health indicators have previously focused on morbidity, mortality, complications and re-admissions. Many operate on the assumption that if resources are available (structural elements) and processes of care seem appropriate, the satisfactory outcomes will be achieved. Examples of these performance indicators include number of pressure sores, hospital acquired infection and re-admission within 30 days. Some are currently being used as Charter Standards and yardsticks in contract monitoring by health care purchasers. (The concept of outcome measures will be discussed further on in this chapter.)

The development of outcomes is also consistent with the desire and need to determine health care priorities and demonstrate the various professionals' contribution to care. Fundamental to any audit approach is the need to establish appropriate criteria against which to measure actual achievement. This requires the development and measurement (usually) of those criteria by experts, people who are familiar with the field in question. The measurement of data for audit can be conducted by non-professionals/other disciplines when methods such as criteria-based audit are used. However, the development of the criteria and technique for measuring must be directed by the relevant professionals. (Criteria-based audit is described later in this chapter.)

Given the complexity and qualitative nature of health care, much of audit relies on soft data, reflective of professional interaction with patients. Therefore, not all elements can be reduced to numerical responses and yes/no answers require an element of interpretation. This interpretation, to be consistent, presupposes an understanding and shared perception by the person auditing the data of the thought processes and intentions of those setting the criteria. It is not surprising, therefore, that the central role of the professionals measuring their own and each other's performance, prevails. Professionals are used to the notion of monitoring their own and their colleagues' performance so the concept of peer review is not unfamiliar to them.

Peer review

A key issue in audit is the question of who sets the standards and evaluates the quality. Medicine has, until recently, been firmly convinced that only doctors can review doctors' work. This view was supported by the Australian Hospital Association (1978) in a monograph which stated that 'the patient is not equipped to judge the professional aspects of medical care, nor the competence of health professionals'. Furthermore it advocated that 'it is not right for (health authorities and Government) to interfere in the professional aspects of medical care.'

It could be argued that these premises are being challenged in the current move to patient centred multidisciplinary clinical audit and consumer satisfaction surveys. However, the principle of peer review is still central to successful audit as specific professions will be more comfortable with scrutinising their own practice before inviting other professional groups to do so.

Peer review is seen by some as a hallmark of professionalism (Passos, 1973) and described by Maas and Jacox (1977) as necessary for demonstrating accountability for practice. In its simplest form, peer review can be used informally by groups to discuss care and how it is organised, or in seeking advice and consultancy from colleagues in other areas. More formal systems would include the setting of standards for care and devising a system for monitoring their achievement. The example of chart audit is a useful illustration of peer review mechanisms. The group decides what elements should be reviewed and sets standards with criteria for ease of measurement. The inclusion of all staff encourages ownership and commitment to the strategy so that subsequent monitoring and plans for change will be willingly accepted.

Most definitions imply that peer review is an activity done by people of the same rank, or equal to one another in status and from the same professional group. This is appropriate when considering aspects of performance in relation to processes of care which can be discreetly identified as the sole domain of one group. When measuring outcomes, however, the edges become blurred and the need for peer review by a multiprofessional group whose 'sameness' is knowledge and expertise in a given speciality should be considered. Collaborative care planning is a good example of the move towards audit by interprofessional peer review.

Common approaches to audit

Meisenheimer (1985) describes audit as structured formal evaluation study based on medical records. This is a narrow perspective and can be widened to embrace observation of practice in some instances. Audit is distinguished by two dimensions, time frame and focus of evaluation. Time frame for audit is the phase in patient care in which data retrieval begins; it can be prospective, concurrent or retrospective.

Prospective review

Prospective review is considered to be a paradox in that care cannot be evaluated before it is given. However, the technique pertains to case identification where the topic for study is selected and cases are recorded from that point forward (e.g. log the next 30 patients with a given diagnosis). These patients become the audit sample. Once the cases have been identified they can be evaluated concurrently or retrospectively. This technique ensures immediacy and accuracy of case identification and economy of time which would otherwise be spent tracking records of patients with a particular diagnosis after discharge.

Meisenheimer considers this prospective approach useful for evaluating nursing/therapy care topics which are not retrievable via standard medical diagnostic coding systems. It could also be used to review high-cost, high-risk cases, e.g. elderly undergoing major cardiac or abdominal surgery, or A&E categories such as suturing of facial wounds, treatment of laceration to hands, or tendon injuries, each of which have potentially significant impact on the patient's future quality of life.

Concurrent review

Concurrent review is considered to be open audit as it takes place while the patient is still receiving care. This term now reflects any quality assurance (QA) evaluation carried out while care is underway. A variety of methods can be used including chart or note review, observation of care delivery and patient and staff interviews. Examples of methods used in nursing include QUALPACS, Slater Rating Scale and Rush Medicus. Each of these American systems can be modified to suit any professional group. The advantages of concurrent audit are:

1. Opportunity to intervene in care where serious deficiencies are discovered. This element highlights one key difference between audit and research where intervention in the latter is avoided unless life threatening professional negligence is observed.
2. Ease and accuracy of audit itself are not limited to what remains of care after the fact (patient memory or case notes).

Retrospective review

Retrospective audit is evaluation after an episode of care is finished. It is typified by comparing predetermined criteria against documentation in charts and case notes. An example of this is the Phaneuf (1976) Nursing Audit. This is a process orientated audit schedule which appraises nursing care as reflected in the patients' records. The principles of this have been used in subsequent developments and again could be modified for other professional groups. Retrospective audit of care may be achieved through patient interviews or post-discharge surveys of satisfaction. Interviews may take place on discharge or at follow up clinic visits, or by use of postal or telephone questionnaire, the effectiveness of the latter being determined by facets of the group being interviewed and the ability of the data collector to communicate well by telephone. The advantages of retrospective audit are the ability to review large numbers of patients and/or their documents. The weakness of retrospective document audit is that certain things are more likely to have been recorded, e.g. physical care or status. This is determined by the perceived purpose of the record:

1. Is it designed to supply enough information to facilitate care? *or*
2. Does it conform to evaluators' expectations and state what was done, when was it done, how was it done and what happened to the patient as a result?

The latter is unlikely to be found in most records; otherwise the recent publication of a learning package on nursing records (NHSTD, 1993), published in response to criticisms from the Ombudsman, would not have been necessary. This learning pack, although prepared for nursing, addresses issues that are relevant to medical and therapy professionals.

The relationship between quality of documentation and quality of care must also be questioned. The correlation is likely to be low and we should beware of making the assumption that if care is charted it has been given or conversely if it is not charted it has not been given.

The limitation of retrospective audit is that it depends largely on the accuracy of the case notes as a reliable record of the episode of care after the event, unless patient surveys of the same clients are undertaken simultaneously. This would provide some balance between staff and patient perspectives. It should be remembered that patients' recollections of recent events will be clearer than earlier intensive periods of care. Significance of events also differs in that patients' main concerns are likely to be about privacy, dignity and interpersonal relationships with staff. Staff, however, usually focus on the resources available to give good care, e.g. physical environment and equipment.

Focus of evaluation of audit

Focus of evaluation for audit includes consideration of structure, process and outcomes.

Structure – all elements creating the environment of care.

Process – all elements involved in professional delivery of care.

Outcome – all elements demonstrating results of care.

In clinical audit, the focus of evaluation is shifting from emphasis on structure and process elements to outcome measures. The assumption that if structure and process seem appropriate, satisfactory outcomes will be inevitable has been challenged and the primacy of a single profession's contribution to, and review of, practice is receding. A recent policy statement from the Department of Health Clinical Outcomes Group (1993) sets the scene for the future integrated multiprofessional approach to clinical audit and outcome measures in particular.

The methods which will be described in this section of the chapter reflect that move towards integration and while some methods were developed for a single profession's use, all are flexible and robust enough to achieve broader application. Methods selected by the medical profession have to date focused on screening of 'events' rather than setting standards, which has been the main focus for nursing and therapy professions. A variety of techniques will be described briefly. as these tend to highlight trends or problem patterns, whereas the remaining methods provide targets for achievement based on professional judgement. These synopses are drawn from the Joint Centre for Medical Education's 1992 publication *Making Medical Audit Effective*.

Adverse event screening

This works on the theory that it may be hard to define what quality is, but we all know what quality is not (JCEM, 1992). Adverse event screening looks at things that should happen, but didn't, or things that shouldn't happen, but did. Events that are not a natural consequence of the disease process or treatment are considered, e.g. medication errors, acute stroke after surgery, pressure sores. This method is more helpful and is used as concurrent audit, i.e. while the patient is in hospital or still being cared for in the community (less easy in general practice).

Critical events

Speciality-specific critical event screening is the systematic monitoring of patients for serious clinical problems which one would always want to evaluate, e.g. post-operative death, unplanned returns to theatre, infection from blood transfusion. These are often described as 'sentinel events' which have a great degree of risk, including medico-legal, attached to them. The advantage of monitoring these events is that they can highlight trends and patterns of identified problems or known risk. Having established the 'problem', investigation takes place into identifying likely causes and action relates to implementing change to minimise future risk.

Advantages:

● Method can be applied universally.
● Alerting mechanism for clinicians/management.

- Adaptable to fit specialities/local requirements.
- Use for multidisciplinary audit.
- Supply management with information without details of individual clinical practice.
- Economical in time and cost; can be performed by non-medical screeners in the first instance.
- Used to identify patterns and trends concurrent or retrospective.

Disadvantages

- Alerting mechanism only – records identified need to be audited subsequently (by review).
- Colleagues may feel threatened by it and fear victimisation.
- Mostly concerns negative outcomes which can raise defences.
- Computer packages available from major companies (expensive).

This system of event screening is a useful method for risk management in relation to clinical practice and could constitute a valuable component of the quality alerting mechanism in the early stages of audit development. Once trends and problems are identified and investigated, standards need to be developed and change implemented. Criteria based audit then becomes the strategy for subsequent review (Joint Centre for Education in Medicine, 1992).

Criteria based audit

The concept of criteria based audit is a popular one and has been developed significantly by nurses over the past eight years. Its development includes:

- Selection of the topic for review.
- Identification of measurable criteria.
- Defining/setting the standard for the aspects of care under consideration.
- Compiling the audit tool and method for data collection.

The standards and criteria are set by the process of group discussion, review of professional publications/guidelines, and review of research literature. The number of criteria identified for each standard can vary enormously but most authors advise a preference for 4–5 with a maximum of 15. Criteria should be stated clearly and succinctly, requiring a single yes/no or numerical response for ease of analysis.

One system for testing the robustness of criteria is to apply the RCN (DySSSy) Standards of Care Project RUMBA mnemonic.

R – Reliable
U – Understandable

M – Measurable
B – Behavioural
A – Acceptable
(Kitson *et al*, 1990)

Having established the standard, criteria and audit tool, the next step is to collect patient data, e.g. case notes, charts, etc. Actual care can then be compared against the pre-set protocols/standards document.

Criteria based audit enables cases to be reviewed and those that fail to meet the standards are identified. Following clinical discussion, changes can be defined and implemented according to an agreed action plan. Further review is then planned using the same criteria applied to a similar group of patients.

Advantages:

● Quality is explicitly expressed and agreed.
● Makes actual practice explicit.
● Audit can be repeated – completing the cycle.
● Concurrent audit enables fast data collection.
● Convergence of practice into agreed standards can be achieved.
● Improvements can be measured.
● Requires explicit statement of local policy.
● Screeners can be non-medical.

Disadvantages:

● Requires accurate clinical indices and information systems.
● Agreeing standards can be difficult and a slow process.
● May require review of a large number of case notes.
● Difficult and time consuming if done by one person retrospectively.
(JCEM, 1992)

Collaborative care planning

Collaborative care planning (CCP) is a multidisciplinary team approach to assessing, planning, implementing and evaluating care in collaboration with the patient, and is developed around an anticipated length of hospital stay or episode of care. This contrasts with the more traditional approach where each discipline plans care in partial or total isolation from others (Finnegan, 1991). The purpose of collaborative care planning is described as making more effective use of resources by ensuring that quality of care is clearly defined, planned, implemented, monitored and audited.

Collaborative care planning (CCP) marks a significant step forward in generating multiprofessional patient focused care with clarity of documentation which enables effective audit. It has become an increasingly popular method since the introduction of QA and patient focused drive by the Department of Health to establish measurable outcomes of care. The idea of multiprofessional debate and decision making is not new to elderly care and psychiatry though much was restricted to verbal discussion and agreement. West Midlands Regional Health Authority, as part of their resource management strategy, set up a major project in six clinical areas. The professional groups had to decide core outcomes of care, critical care paths using flow charts and a single plan of care with each profession's input clearly defined (towards the common goal).

The advantages of CCP, described by the West Midlands Regional Health Authority (Finnegan, 1991) in the project report, are congruence of purpose, clarification of complementary interventions and reductions in repetitive intervention, task overlap and confusion or omissions. CCP provides a clear set of records/data for audit purposes with care that has been validated between professions. Audit is conducted concurrently, with hourly or daily monitoring of care plans but retrospective audit would also be more reliable in the presence of such comprehensive care planning and consistency of documentation.

Appendix 3 is an example of a collaborative care plan for cholecystectomy from Burton Hospital NHS Trust (1991). It demonstrates not only the integration of multiprofessional care in the acute hospital setting but also the move towards 'seamless care' on discharge to the community care setting. CCP has management benefits in that it provides information for costing care, measuring the quality and supporting case mix analyses. The process contributes to the monitoring of contracts of care through its provision of explicit information of what is intended and what has been achieved. Collaborative care planning documentation can include detailed care plans as illustrated, but also flow charts indicating key stages of care that must be achieved as part of the expected route to recovery. Such charts of key events have been developed in various guises:

Critical paths
Anticipated recovery paths
Care maps
Care profiles

Critical path analysis

The flow charts generated in the CCP are a form of critical path analysis. It is a technique for analysing a process in terms of activities and events that must be completed in a specified sequence in order to achieve a goal. Some activities can be done concurrently while others can only commence when another activity is completed. In developing critical paths it is necessary to identify:

1. The components of the recovery/care episode.
2. The time required for each.
3. The sequence of events to achieve the desired outcome.

From a variety of options the 'critical path' is identified or selected.

Critical care paths evolved as part of managed care in the USA and are integral to case mix management for resource management initiatives. The critical path is a condensed flow chart depicting key sequential events and expected progress through the episode of care. Deviations from the planned care can be identified at a glance, enabling corrective action to be taken. The 'deviations' from planned care are recorded, investigated (as necessary) and analysed, and appropriate corrective interventions are decided and implemented. This is known as 'Variance Analysis'.

The value and benefit of critical path analysis is that the content provides objective and relevant data for clinical audit, while providing information to guide care delivery, monitor case mix management and resource use. Ownership of the critical path is important and should be shared by medical, nursing and therapy professionals. Clarity of each discipline's contribution helps identify the most appropriate coordinator of care, based on level of contribution and significance of, or responsibility for, key decision taking. Initially it may be appropriate for medical staff to take the lead in acute medical and surgical areas. The rapidity of change and uncertainty of response demands a high level of medical decision in the early stages of diagnosis and management. Once daily 'doctoring' is no longer required, then rehabilitation, maintenance care and palliative care are probably best managed/led by nursing or therapy professionals.

Care maps

Care maps are another tool of case management. They show critical or key incidents that must occur in a predictable and timely fashion to achieve appropriate length of stay in hospital. It can be seen from this description that care maps are similar to critical paths and anticipated recovery paths.

Addenbrooke's Hospital, Cambridge, has adopted care maps as a vehicle for case management and clinical audit. The care maps have been compiled by a multidisciplinary group, helped by the care map facilitator who is a senior nurse manager. The care maps have a uniform grid structure with eight sections – consultations, tests, treatments, medications, diet, activity, teaching, discharge, planning – cross-divided by the anticipated number of days of treatment. Anticipated interventions are logged onto the grid. In addition to the individual patient administration details, care maps include:

Names of compiling group.
Review date.
Case type (including ICD Code).
LoS (length of stay).

Appendix 4 is an example of a care map for myocardial infarction from Addenbrooke's NHS Trust (1992). The care map is reviewed, variances identified and checked against predetermined codes. Variances are analysed monthly by the compiling group and the resultant data assist the case mix management group to identify causes of variance and collectively to determine changes to practice/service. The tool itself is also reviewed every six months.

In practical terms, care maps describe when various activities should occur, e.g. when patient assessment is performed, discharge plan completed, antibiotic therapy stops or wound drains removed. A designated person, ward sister or senior professional checks if the activity was performed and notes the reason on a variance chart if it was not done in the specified time. Care maps, therefore, form a standard against which care given is compared. The variance analysis and care map review can provide data for both concurrent and retrospective audit.

Care profiles

Care profiles are yet another tool of case mix management systems and provide a retrospective method for comparing treatment profiles against actual care given. Care profiles in the UK originated in Huddersfield (Sainsbury, 1991) as part of the resource management (RM) initiative. The philosophy of RM advocates that the clinical information system should handle standards of care and be owned by individual consultants. In aggregating profiles of care derived from individual consultants, different working practices become evident. With common conditions it is reasonable to expect to set a consistent profile. Sainsbury anticipates that 80% of a surgeon's workload could be covered by 24 profiles. He acknowledges that 92% of his own operating was done within 27 operation codes. Although physicians may argue this is a more complex and disparate workload, consistency is still feasible for many conditions, e.g. myocardial infarction, diabetes, epilepsy, ulcerative colitis, etc.

Profiles of care, like care maps and critical paths, can form the basis for medical and clinical audit if established by a multidisciplinary group. Profiles of care as developed from a medical perspective consist of:

- Minimum expected and maximum length of stay.
- Mortality rate for a particular diagnosis.
- Number and type of tests.
- Operations and likely complications that may occur.

As with other techniques, actual practice is compared against the set profile of care. Profiles have been used in retrospective criterion based audit, and fit well into the audit cycle.

- Profile of care established for topic.
- Profile comparison performed (actual v expected).
- Standards set/implemented.
- Data gathered for further comparison.
- Change implemented (either profile, practice or both).

All of these techniques can be manually driven, e.g. paper exercises, or computerised (depending on availability of IT/suitable systems), or a combination of both.

The basis for critical paths, care maps, ARPs, CCP and profiles of care, are usually medical diagnostic categories/codes (ICD), e.g. myocardial infarction, cholecystectomy. The tools therefore relate to patient groupings rather than individual patient needs assessment. Symptom-generated protocols would be required for ensuring individualised patient profiles/map etc., but as the majority of cases fall into a limited number of diagnostic categories and respond similarly, individualisation at the outset would seem unnecessary. Individualisation of care would, therefore, be determined by:

a) Patient assessment recognising the need for amendment and integration of protocols in the face of multi-pathology;
b) Analysis of variance as occurs from standard protocol, responses being 'tailored' to the individual patient's need.

Ownership by the multidisciplinary team and patient involvement appear to be strong threads in using care protocols (profiles, maps, ARPs, CCP). Most authors/users advocate the sharing of information and decision making with the client/patient and encourage the location of protocols at the bedside, thus enhancing joint evaluation of care.

Off the shelf packages

Various audit packages have been mentioned, which while developed for nursing could be modified for use by other professions.

Phaneuf nursing audit

The audit tool identifies 50 components of nursing care from seven key functions and focuses attention on the patient rather than the specialities of the nurses who give the care. The components are stated in terms of actions by nurses in relation to the patient and in the form of questions to be answered by the reviewer as they look back at the patient's record. A numerical score is derived from the results and equated with five statements – excellent, good, incomplete, poor, unsafe (Phaneuf, 1976).

QUALPACS

This tool was designed to measure the standard of nursing care received by a patient or group of patients. A derivation of the Slater Nursing Performance Scale, used widely in the USA. QUALPACS (Wandelt and Ager, 1974) evaluates the performance of an individual nurse as she is observed giving care. Performance is measured against a given standard on a five-point scale which is then scored and aggregated to give an overall score. QUALPACS can be used in any care setting where nurses interact with clients and observation periods last more than two and a half hours. The QUALPACS schedule includes 68 elements of care classified in six broad headings addressing physical, psychosocial, general, communication and professional implications. Again the performance is rated numerically and results in an overall score. The pitfall of QUALPACS is the complexity of the schedule, attempting to record all observations against the 68 items can be difficult and may result in omissions or errors. However, the principle of the system is sound and a simplified version has much to offer when developing tools for measuring processes of care.

Process or outcome measures

The focus on outcome measures of health care is a natural progression in the quest for quality. The effectiveness of health care and professional services should be determined by results – evidence of change in health status in relation to predetermined targets. In the climate dominated by concern for 'value for money', critical review and limited resources, there is a need to demonstrate that professional inputs result in beneficial outcomes for patients.

The identification and assessment of outcomes is a key component of the NHS reforms, to be achieved through the audit process. Nursing should be acknowledged for leading the movement in establishing care standards with the work of the RCN Standards of Care Programme. *The Dynamic*

Standard Setting System (DySSSy) developed by Kitson (1990) has been widely acclaimed by nurses across the country. The use of Donabedian's Structure–Process–Outcome framework for generating criteria has in itself encouraged people to focus on tangible, measurable patient centred outcomes within the standard setting exercise.

Outcome measures have been postulated as the key to establishing cost effectiveness of care but Bond (1993) questions if they can stand alone. She proposes that if the concern is solely 'what good are we doing?' then it could be argued that the end result is sufficient evidence regardless of how it was achieved. Bond believes that we need to establish outcomes in relation to processes of care, i.e. matching or demonstrating relationships between the two. This would provide substantiated evidence of the results of care and allow recognition of tortuous paths to recovery which do not constitute cost effectiveness or good value for money.

Outcomes are best stated in patient terms as this allows for the influence of all disciplines involved in the care of a given patient. The appropriateness of outcomes must be considered in situations like death or chronic illness where recovery or improvement in health status is unlikely. Bond (1991) suggests that emphasis on outcome measures in these instances would focus on satisfaction with care, reduction of symptoms, quality of survival or maintenance of steady state. The relationship between process and outcomes is an important element in such situations as the majority of consumers fall into the acute on chronic category of illness. Bond is currently coordinating research into outcomes of nursing care at the Centre for Health Services Research, University of Newcastle upon Tyne. The three year research project was commissioned by the Department of Health in 1991 as one of the funded projects in nursing and therapy clinical audit. One aspect of the research is to test the sensitivity of instruments supposed to measure *nursing* outcomes. Three conditions were selected to analyse outcome measures – hysterectomy, myocardial infarction and fractured neck of femur. Each of these is seen as having a high nursing component and therefore outcomes could be reflective of nursing's specific contribution.

Outcome measures currently available include morbidity and mortality statistics, complications, readmission rates (though the latter are acknowledged to be inaccurate) and patient satisfaction. Clare (1990) argues it is indefensible to avoid measures of outcome and rely on measures of 'output' merely because the tools are lacking or crude. Existing measures should be used to improve care until, through experience and increasing expertise, better and more direct measures become available. Future outcome measures must recognise the influence of various factors. Clare suggests that anthropologists should be involved as culture, social background, patient attitude as well as availability of medical resources impact on outcomes. Several centres have taken up the challenge and we are undertaking work on establishing outcome measures. The Department of Health has established a national clearing house for assessing health service outcomes, at the Nuffield Institute for Health Services, Leeds University (Long, 1992). Much of the work being done is geared to developing improved methods for measuring clinical outcomes in relation to functional health status perceptions of health and severity of illness.

The appropriateness of the timing of outcome measurement has to be considered, as Hardwick (1992) discovered. Hardwick and his colleagues undertook a study in Taunton, monitoring outcomes after discharge from the surgical unit. They highlighted an unrecognised incidence of post-operative infection following appendicectomy because of early discharge from hospital.

The measurement phase

The measurement of response to health care intervention is of critical importance in judging the beneficial or adverse effects on patients. Many sytems for measuring and evaluating care and sources of data are readily available to the health professional in the workplace. Patients are a primary source of data. Observation of their behaviour, emotional and physiological, can provide powerful evidence of their response to illness and care interventions, e.g. response to analgesia, indicating the efficiency of pain relief. Questioning patients about the effectiveness of pain relief can also be useful, though some patients may 'pretend' to feel better because that's what they think staff want to hear.

Pain measurement scales

These are a useful adjunct to evaluating both intensity or relief of pain. Although subjective assessments, as they rely on the patient perception, pain measurement scales can be sensitive and reproducible (McQuay, 1990). Scales differ for measuring intensity of pain or pain relief. Both visual analogue and categorical scales are available.

Visual analogue
These are often depicted as horizontal lines with end markers. Patients indicate a point along the line which corresponds to their perception of the relief achieved, or intensity of pain experienced. Pain 'thermometer' scales have also been developed which offer fixed markings or points between the two extremes. Some people question the influence or orientation of intermediate line markings, especially if the intermittent markings categorise the level of pain. Categorical scales are usually less popular as they force

Relief of pain

No   — — — — — — — — — — — — — — —   Complete
relief   relief

Intensity of pain

Least   — — — — — — — — — — — — — —   Worst
possible   possible
pain   pain

the patient to choose from a fixed selection of phrases, none of which may reflect his perception at the time. For example:

Intensity of Pain	*Relief*
Severe	Complete
Moderate	Good
Slight	Moderate
None	Slight
	None

Patients are asked to tick against the most appropriate statement. Pain charts facilitate the monitoring of pain intensity and/or relief over a period of time and provide trends indicating effectiveness and duration of pain control. They therefore have a useful role as data for clinical audit purposes.

There are numerous measurement scales available for monitoring **functional ability** (e.g. Barthel Index), health status (Nottingham Health Profile), psychological well-being, social networks and social support and life satisfaction and morale. A comprehensive review of a number of these has been compiled by Bowling (1991).

Barthel Index

The scale depicting functional ability is well used by the therapy professions when assessing the elderly or stroke patients. It covers nine dimensions:

Feeding.
Mobility from bed to chair.
Personal toilet (washing, etc.).
Getting on/off the toilet.
Bathing.
Walking on level surface.
Gong up/down stairs.
Dressing.
Incontinence (bladder and bowel).

Designed by Mahoney and Barthel (1965) it is based on observed functions and developed to measure functional ability before and after intervention treatment and to indicate the amount of care required. Although designed for use with long-term patients with neuromuscular and skeletal disorders, it has been used more generally. The index was originally designed for hospital use but has been extended to include activities of daily living and therefore its area of applicability has widened. The patient is scored on 10 activities which are summed to give an overall score between 0 (totally dependent) and 100 (fully independent).

The Barthel Index is popular, especially in care of the elderly and stroke units, although Bowling (1991) urges caution, claiming that while its simplicity is an attraction, it also poses major limitations on its use and that further testing is required before its use could be recommended. For the purposes of clinical audit, the Barthel Index can make a useful contribution as one of a range of scales used in monitoring outcomes of some groups of patients with limited functional ability.

Nottingham Health Profile

The NHP was developed by Hunt *et al* (1986) in the UK and is based on lay perceptions of health. It is not an index of disease, illness or disability but relates to how people feel when experiencing different states of health (Bowling, 1991). The profile was developed after interviews with a large number of lay people about the effects of illness on behaviour. Bowling describes the NHP as a useful survey tool in assessing whether people have a (severe) health problem at all, but diagnostic data would be required to identify the kind of health problem. The NHP is concise and designed for self completion. It has been widely used in the UK and abroad, tested for validity and partly for reliability across a range of patient groups, including pregnant women, rheumatoid arthritis sufferers, people with fractures and heart and lung transplants.

The NHP is in two parts and covers six areas in Part I – physical mobility, pain, sleep, energy, emotional reactions and social isolation. There are 38 statements requiring yes/no responses, and possible scores of 0–100. Part II asks about effects of health on seven areas of daily life – work, looking after the home, social life, home life, sex life, interests, hobbies and holidays. These are also coded for yes/no answers and scored. As can be seen, some items would not necessarily be relevant to certain groups, e.g. elderly, unemployed, disabled, low income people. The authors have acknowledged the limitations of Part II, and advise against its use until further developmental work has been completed.

Case notes

Measurement scales are one useful source of data, especially for capturing patient perception, but other sources, including case notes and charts, are equally valuable in monitoring care. As mentioned earlier in this chapter, case notes can be used for concurrent and retrospective audit. The content of case notes can be scrutinised against a criterion checklist to measure the adequacy and accuracy of patient or clinical information. Case notes data can be used to confirm or refute appropriateness of care prescribed, observed and/or given. However, in order to do this, the reliability of the case notes must not be in doubt. Clinical observation charts also contribute to the sources of data available for audit, especially surgical wound assessment, infection surveillance charts.

The measurement tools and sources described so far are related to direct clinical care, but there is another important area for measurement, and that is the appropriateness and quality of the environment in which care is given. Health and safety is an essential element in the clinical care arena as unrecognised or ignored hazards can adversely affect both patients and staff. Health and safety monitoring and inspection can be integrated with, or an adjunct to, clinical audit.

Verbal feedback

One of the most effective ways of gathering information is to ask. Patients, relatives and staff can provide varied and invaluable feedback as to the effectiveness of care. How to ask for information becomes less simple and straightforward. The choice between using interview or questionnaire needs to be considered.

Interviews

Interviews can be conducted formally or informally, with the interview following a rigorous schedule (often a questionnaire) or inviting open comments. The value of following a prescriptive schedule or questionnaire is one of speed and consistency, though this may be at the expense of the quality of the data. Prescriptive schedules ask only the questions listed, and therefore limit the range of responses, whereas an informal discussion seeking patients' or relatives' perceptions about their stay/contact with the care environment, may elicit unexpected areas of information and aspects of concern. Interviews also allow for clarification and expansion of questions and responses which can enhance the quality and quantity of information received. Interviews are not without drawbacks; use of language, especially 'medical' jargon, can bias responses as can body language and environment.

Questionnaires

Questionnaires are often considered an easy option for gathering opinions. They certainly allow large numbers of people to be surveyed, but the style, length and use of language again can have an adverse effect and bias responses. Questionnaires must be carefully designed and rigorously piloted on a group of people similar to the proposed population to be surveyed. There are no opportunities to clarify or expand on the content of questionnaires if sent through the post or left with people to self-administer. Questionnaires can include a range of forced choice or closed questions which require yes/no or tick box responses. These are easy to analyse, but restrictive in that responses are limited to the choices made available. Questionnaires which include open questions (e.g. 'What did you like most about your stay in hospital? ') allow for a free response and will generate a variety of unexpected comments which are complex and time consuming to analyse.

Observation

Another technique which can be used is 'observation'. Observation of clinical practice can provide valuable insight into what staff and/or patients do. Observing staff provides another dimension to asking their opinions or reviewing case records and enables comparison of actual practice against prescribed or expected care. Observation of practice can be very valuable in monitoring both processes and outcomes of care. A variety of research techniques can be used to observe practice, including non participation where the observer has no involvement in activity other than to record what is seen. This can pose an ethical and moral dilemma for the observer if they witness care or practices which are detrimental to the patients' safety. Unlike a research activity there is no reason in audit for the observer to stand back. They should be at liberty to act as necessary as long as the episode is clearly recorded for future discussion and action. Observation can take place using a predetermined set of criteria against which to measure activity, e.g. QUALPACS. The familiarity and proficiency of the observers must be considered as should the need for consistency if two or more observers will be monitoring the same area. If the observation schedule is robust enough it may be preferable to use an observer who can bring a fresh eye to the proceedings. Other observation techniques can include the use of a 'mystery shopper', someone unfamiliar to the staff and area who tests the service.

Summary

This chapter has attempted to give an overview of audit methodologies and to illustrate some examples which have particular value in clinical audit. Consideration has been given to the focus and timing of audit activity as well as how it may be done. Reference has been made to well established techniques which it is felt could be adapted for use by nursing and the therapy professions, singly or jointly. While by no means detailed or complete, it is hoped that sufficient flavour has been provided to whet the appetite of those currently involved and those about to become involved in audit.

References

Addenbrooke's NHS Trust (1992) *Care Map for Myocardial Infarction*. Cambridge: Addenbrooke's NHS Trust.

Australian Hospital Association (1978) *Peer Review and Cost Containment – An appraisal*. Health Service Monograph No. 1, SP/78.

Bond S (1991) *Outcomes of Hospital Nursing in the Acute Sector*. Discussion paper for the Department of Health. Unpublished.

Bowling A (1991) *Measuring Health: A review of quality of life measurement scales*. Milton Keynes: Open University Press.

Burton Hospital NHS Trust (1991) *Collaborative Care Plan for Cholecystectomy*. Burton Hospital NHS Trust.

Clare A (1990) In A Hopkins and D Costain (eds) *Measuring the Outcomes of Medical Care*. London Royal College of Physicians and King's Fund Centre for Health Services Development.

Department of Health (1989) *Working for Patients*. London: HMSO.

Department of Health (1992) *Health of the Nation*. London: HMSO.

Department of Health (1993) *Clinical Audit Meeting and Improving Standards in Health Care*. (Clinical Outcomes Group.) London: HMSO.

Donabedian A (1986) Criteria and standards for quality monitoring. *Quality Review Bulletin* **12** (3): 99–100.

Finnegan E (1991) *Collaborative Care Planning. A natural catalyst for change*. Resource Management Support Unit, West Midlands Health Region.

Goldstone L, Ball J, Collier M (1983) *Monitor: An Index of the Quality of Nursing Care for Acute Medical and Surgical Wards*. Newcastle upon Tyne Polytechnic Products Ltd.

Hardwick R, Saltrese-Taylor A and Collins C (1992) Need to measure outcome after discharge in surgical audit. *Quality in Health Care* **1** (3): 165–167.

Hunt S, McEwan J, McKenna S (1986) *Measuring Health Status*. London: Croom Helm.

Joint Centre for Education in Medicine (1992) *Making Medical Audit Effective*. Module 3: Methods of Audit. London: JCEM.

King's Fund Centre (1990) *Organisational Audit Project*, London: King's Fund.

Kitson A, Hyndman S, Harvey G and Yerrell P (1990) *Quality Patient Care: The Dynamic Standard Setting System*. London: Scutari Press.

Maas M and Jacox A (1977) *Guidelines for Nurse Autonomy/Patient Welfare*. New York: Appleton-Century-Crofts.

Mahoney F and Barthel D (1965) Cited in A Bowling (1991) *Measuring Health*. Milton Keynes: Open University Press.

McQuay H (1989) In A Hopkins and D Costain (eds) (1990) *Measuring the Outcomes of Medical Care*. London: Royal College of Physicians and King's Fund Centre for Health Service Development.

Meisenheimer C (1985) *Quality Assurance: A Complete Guide to Effective Programs*. Maryland, USA: Aspen Publications.

National Health Services Training Directorate (1992) *Keeping the Records Straight*. Bristol: NHSTD.

Passos J (1973) Cited in A Pearson (ed) (1987) *Nursing Quality Measurement: Quality Assurance Methods for Peer Review*. Chichester: John Wiley & Sons.

Phaneuf M (1974) *The Nursing Audit*. New York: Appleton-Century-Crofts.

Sainsbury R, Freer J and Brennan S (1991) *Profiles of Care and their Influence on Surgical Audit*. Paper presented at Clinical Profiles of Care Workshop, March 1991. NHS Management Executive. Petersfield: Status.

Wandelt M and Ager J (1974) *Quality Patient Care Scale*. New York: Appleton-Century-Crofts.

4

Linking Resource Management, Quality and Audit

Background

Audit could be seen as yet another 'initiative' from the 'centre' (Department of Health), which affects those providers who become caught up with the idea, and leaves others untouched and unscathed. Previous initiatives such as total quality management and resource management, like audit, have represented large sums of money for providers in the form of pump priming to achieve the strategic goals of the initiative. This money tends to be distributed from the centre or its agents (e.g. regional health authorities), in response to bids from purchasers or providers. Such project or flexible income is vital to the development of the provider and contributes greatly to the provider's image within the NHS and with the public. Providers become flagships for different initiatives, giving them status on NHS conference platforms and providing good publicity locally. The biggest danger of such initiatives is that they are often supported to the neglect of other equally vital issues, becoming an end in themselves rather than the process to achieve an end. They become self-perpetuating and dominant within the Trust, rather than assuming a supportive role to the Trust's overall development. Moreover, the fact that they become an important source of income and the most important investment for the provider unit can mean that other initiatives become of secondary importance, and may grow in isolation. This is particularly so in the case of resource management and quality where whole career structures now exist with explicit roles to support the initiative, with staff becoming 'quality' experts. While this may seem desirable, the tendency can be for those staff to bury themselves within the particular initiative, concentrating on delivering that one sphere of health service management without coming up for air and ensuring that they are still within sight of land.

Thus in sites that have championed resource management, the danger has been that audit is seen as a separate initiative, requiring separate management systems to implement it and separate information technology to resource it. Certainly at the inception of audit, it would have been dangerous to attempt to link audit to other performance systems such as resource management, as the doctors who believed that audit was their professional territory and were prone to scepticism on its value, could well have refused to participate in the audit process. This is reflected in a study into doctors' attitudes to audit, undertaken by the Health Service Research Unit, at the London School of Hygiene and Tropical Medicine, which demonstrates that, in general, doctors are at best ambivalent about the value of audit (Black and Thompson, 1993).

Thus, separate funding of audit, quality, resource management and research and development has reinforced the separateness of these initiatives. In truth they are wholly interdependent, and require a coordinated strategy within each provider unit.

Resource management

The main thrust of the resource management initiative (RM) was to involve clinicians (meaning doctors) in management to attempt to ensure that those who were responsible for the majority of resource use and thus allocation, actually held that responsibility managerially. The aim of resource management was to improve the service to patients by enabling resource allocation decisions to take place, based on sound information about the impact of that allocation on the service as a whole. This impact evaluation is the concern of organisational audit (see Chapter 3) and clinical audit. However, at the inception of RM, neither of these audit processes was taking place systematically, nor was there the expertise available within clinical directorates to make sense of the information that was being generated. Systematic evaluation of clinical care and the care management process was a vital missing component.

Packwood *et al* (1991) have identified four interrelated factors within RM:

> *Improved quality of care* as a result of the service providers, the doctors, nurses and paramedics who directly treat and care for patients, having direct access to information about the effectiveness of different patterns of treatment and greater authority to determine the deployment of resources.

> *Involvement in management by the service providers* whose decisions directly commit resources to patient treatment and care.

> *Improved information* to identify how resources are being used, with what effect and what are the alternatives.

Stronger control of resources that results from rational and responsible management and use of information, for resource allocation and determining service activities.

The language of evaluation, review and quality improvement features strongly within these factors, demonstrating the interrelationships with quality and audit. The factors identified had two practical manifestations within the RM process – development of new management structures and development of information technology to support those structures.

a) *Management structures*
The resource management initiative was seen as the same as the clinical directorate management structure, with doctors as the clinical directors for a cohort of clinical services. The clinical director controls the total budget (minus some support services) for that directorate and is responsible for the performance of that directorate to the chief executive and Trust board. The clinical director is supported by a business manager and/ or a nurse manager. This means that nurses and professions allied to medicine are responsible managerially to the clinical director and professionally to the most senior relevant professional in the organisation (in the case of nursing this is the Trust nurse executive). The desire was to involve doctors more closely in the decisions about resource allocation and management, reflecting the fact that their clinical decisions are pivotal to that process. While some doctors took to the new posts like ducks to water, others shunned the initiative as a waste of their clinical time and expertise. The former tended to be those that were cooperative and active in service management anyway. The latter sought to undermine the process by refusing to become accountable to the clinical director, citing the importance of clinical freedom and personal accountability to the patient to prescribe the best treatment possible in their personal judgement. Where clinical directorates flourish there has been a sense of group identity and multidisciplinary involvement, fostering a willingness to solve problems.

b) *Information technology*
The NHS invested and continues to invest heavily in information technology, in order to track patients through the service and identify where, and on what, resources are used. These systems incorporated, where possible, existing information systems such as the patient administration system and the human resource system. In relation to nursing, the information collected tended to concentrate on the nursing inputs to care, i.e. nursing activity or workload. This was later expanded to incorporate a more individual way of monitoring activity through computerised care planning systems. The focus of data capture has been on inpatient activity, captured in the case mix system which has been dominated by medical

diagnosis. The information requirements tended to pertain to determining the cost of activities, relating that to the volume of work undertaken. The development of the systems concentrated on the medical experiences of the patient, with nursing added on as an afterthought and therapists often ignored completely. This supported the ethos behind the management structures, which was to begin to get a grip on medical decision making and the impact of that on the management of resources. It also assumed, wrongly, that the costs and activity of the other services is dependent on the medical diagnosis. Unfortunately patients are much more complex than a simple medical label.

Thus, the decentralisation of management to clinical directorates and the development of universal data capture and analysis was to lead to informed decision making and greater work identity among the professionals. However, the data capture in many hospitals is still being developed, and community services are only just beginning to be supported in developing their information requirements. With the advent of contracting in the NHS, the information systems became even more vital in providing information on the costs, volume and quality of services. To date, information systems have tended to concentrate on the inputs to the care process, i.e. the resources attributed to a particular activity, with some information on the care process itself (e.g. profiles of care, or activities carried out). This is assessed against productivity and bed occupancy as a measurement of output of the care process. Thus, an efficient service will seek to minimise cost and maximise throughput and bed occupancy without reducing quality or while enhancing quality. Decisions are thus made about the most cost effective use of staff, theatre time, clinical supplies, outpatient sessions and pressure relieving equipment etc.

The overlap between RM and audit becomes apparent, in that audit provides some of the missing links to enable effective decision making by attempting systematically to analyse the actual care and treatment received by the patient. Resource management prior to audit had attempted to make decisions in a vacuum, in that the effectiveness of clinical practices were alluded to, rather than systematically challenged. Some clinicians emphasised that you couldn't make resource decisions without having a notion of the impact those decisions would make on the patient. They developed care profiles as a way of beginning to compare services against accepted norms (see Chapter 3). This pre-empted the central medical audit initiative and demonstrated the timeliness of the arrival of audit. The fact that resource decisions were being made in the absence of any assessment of clinical performance was perhaps the reason that it was so difficult to demonstrate any positive cost benefit analysis of the whole initiative. As with all such initiatives, RM required organisational and professional change to address the fundamentals of practices that hindered service development.

The arrival of audit heralded another plethora of commercial information systems. Clinicians seem easily seduced by information technology and the daunting task of capturing and analysing clinial data meant that many looked for quick fix solutions. However, it is more than obvious that audit should look to those systems already developed to enhance the audit process. Alas, this very development meant that some hospital systems were already out of date. In the case of nursing, they had concentrated on information to support service management (e.g. workload measurement to compare demand and supply in order to rationalise nursing time) or, in some cases, the development of computerised information systems to reduce the waiting time for information related to treatments or tests. Few of these systems attempted to identify the nursing or therapy components of individual patients' experiences. Where this was attempted, it took place in isolation from the system devised to track medical care. The fault could be said to lie in the attempt to simplify inherently complex decisions, and in the attempt to provide information assuming that the organisational development would take place on the back of hard evidence. In truth, it should have happened the other way round. This is being rectified now with the instigation of clinical information systems. However, in order to capture the variety of information requirements related to the patient's whole experience, clinicians must have a say in 'determining the function of any proposed case mix/clinical audit system' (Mosley, 1992). This involvement includes detailed analysis of current and future information requirements and requires some intensive crystal ball gazing. Nursing, while being penalised within RM by the perception that it was an add on luxury, has been more fortunate in adapting to the requirements of audit, in that it could use existing care planning systems to compare the actual care with the standardised plan of care for that particular patient need. The drawback is that this again only captures the process of care without any concern for outcomes. The professions allied to medicine (PAMs) have been relatively isolated in the whole process. Their involvement has been marginal and seen as an add on to any nursing system already available.

Quality

Go to any conference, read any policy statement, pick up any journal and you will find the word quality again and again. Improving the quality of the service has become the *raison d'être* of the NHS manager and professional. This is part of a broader remit to achieve value for money consisting of efficiency, effectiveness and economy. The competition within the managed market of the NHS has driven quality up the agenda so that providers actively market their services on quality, usually in terms of Maxwell's six dimensions (Maxwell, 1984), namely:

Accessibility
Relevance
Effectiveness
Equity
Social acceptability
Efficiency and economy

These quality dimensions are assessed as part of the organisation's quality strategy and criteria related to each are incorporated into the contracts. Commonly, service review takes the form of patient satisfaction through questionnaires which feature these dimensions, e.g. for Accessibility the following question may be asked: 'Do you think that the sign-posting in the hospital is adequate to enable you to find your way about?'

Total quality management

Quality in the NHS has been heavily pump-primed through the total quality management (TQM) initiative. TQM was imported from the Japanese and relies on the following four principles:

1. Organisational success is dependent on meeting the requirements of its customers.
2. Quality is dependent on the processes of production. These have within them complex causal relationships which have to be understood.
3. Employees are intrinsically motivated to do well in their work.
4. Analysis of data related to work processes can lead to insight and understanding of those processes and their causal relationships, leading to improvements. (Berwick *et al*, 1992)

The emphasis in TQM is on process, which it is assumed will lead to better outcomes or outputs. In attempting to meet the requirements of TQM and the analogy that quality is everyone's business, assessments of the quality of the service usually include patient/consumer feedback in some form, and initiatives such as the development of standards, quality circles and diagonal slices incorporating all levels of the organisation. Some Trusts have adopted what they perceive to be the next step in quality, namely, continuous quality improvement (CQI). In reality this is just the American label for TQM (Walshe and Coles, 1993)

Standards

Standard setting based on the Donabedian dimensions of structure, process and outcome (1990) has been developed at all levels of the service but in nursing has been seen primarily as a bottom-up approach (Kitson, 1989).

While commendable in ensuring ownership by clinical staff, this approach has caused difficulties in terms of implementation, as clinical staff seek research based standards without necessarily addressing resource or organisational constraints. It has also caused some difficulties in terms of multidisciplinary delivery and organisational ownership, which causes disillusionment and disappointment. The other hindrance has been the plethora of standards developed and the difficulty in prioritising these, or weighting them in terms of overall importance. Asking staff what they are concerned about, in order to select a topic for standard setting, is neither systematic nor logical. Finally, once developed, monitoring of those standards has tended to take a back seat. This has meant that there has been a tendency for nurses to invest a lot of time and energy in developing standards that could be seen by the organisation as impossible to achieve, which could be viewed by other professionals as low priority and by patients as irrelevant, and which are implemented for a period of months before being assigned to the back of a drawer never to be seen again (or resurrected when the problem recurs in a year's time).

For standards to be meaningful they must be owned by all involved in care delivery, from the clinical nurse to the Trust board; they must be understandable; they must be realistic; they must have an action plan for change and development, based on a realistic timetable; and they must be monitored regularly. It is unlikely that any clinical team can develop and tackle more than six or seven standards in any one year. These standards should be developed from the concerns of patients, the purchasers, the managers and the clinical staff, and should reflect the current research agenda which is generating information on which to develop services or define best practices. These standards should then form part of the audit agenda and a subsequent maintenance monitoring agenda.

The emphasis within quality as a whole has been on the setting up of systems, rather than any monitoring process. However, quality assurance packages have been available for nursing, assessing the quality of care in relation to the process of care and the environment in which care takes place (see Chapter 3). Nursing has taken the lead in quality within many organisations, with quality at organisational board level seen as the remit of the Trust nurse. While this could be seen as a positive role for nursing, in reality it has reflected the overall status of quality in the organisation and has led to quality initiatives primarily involving nurses and general managers, without capturing the interest of doctors or other health care professionals. Thus, doctors are just beginning to discover standard setting on the back of their involvement in audit and do not tend to recognise that this expertise already exists within nursing. Nursing audit packages have originated from this strong involvement in quality assurance, attempting to add a monitoring measurement function to the standard setting process. This has been a simple approach which has denied the developmental work or change part of the audit cycle, concentrating effort on standard setting and measurement. As with most audit mechanisms, the denial of the importance of change facilitation and management means that much valuable time is wasted and expectations dashed.

The link between quality and resources has been championed as part of the reviews of nursing resources. Attempts to standardise nurse staffing patterns for clinical services have seen a plethora of reports. The most recent one, by the York Health Economics Research Group (1992), demonstrated that essentially you get what you pay for, i.e. more qualified nurses = better care outputs. However, standardised packages are coming under increasing scrutiny. *Monitor* (1990), much favoured in the 1980s, is beginning to lose credibility as nurses seek to make relationships between process and outcome, recognising the complexity of the causal relationships identified in TQM. Moreover, such measures seek to standardise the professional's response to individual patients – a concept that still causes reactions of horror among clinicians.

Thus, quality initiatives such as TQM have concentrated on creating an organisational climate for quality, while instigating a range of approaches that seek to marry bottom up and top down. They have created the foundation for audit in the setting of standards within some professional groups, seeking to emphasise quality assurance. Many organisations now view audit as a natural part of their quality strategy. In launching the new approach to clinical audit in 1993, Mrs Moores, director of nursing at the NHS Management Executive, said:

> Although audit is important, it is only one tool in the achievement of continuous quality improvement in delivering patient care.

This signifies a clear direction for audit within a total quality strategy. Audit has obvious links with quality but it also has links with resource management. The challenge is to develop a strategy and approach that builds on the strengths of each of these initiatives, namely:

- Outputs must be considered in the context of inputs.
- Processes of care are dependent on a number of causal factors including human motivation.
- Quality is everyone's business.
- Decentralised decision making will ensure ownership of decisions and action.
- Accurate information is the key to the success of decision making.
- Information does not necessarily lead to change.

The value for money equation

There is no 'body' of literature on the costs and benefits of nursing, but rather a series of often incompatible parts . . . There is a requirement for more UK research which formulates and validates methodologies for measuring cost in relation to outcome. (From *Caring Costs. Nursing Benefits: a review for the Royal College of Nursing*, James Buchan and Jane Ball (1991))

The imperative for nursing in the current managerial climate is to demonstrate the cost benefits of nursing practice. At present, we have studies investigating the effects on patient care and costs of a reduced or increased skill level (Bagust and Burrows, 1992); we have resource management attempting to relate the costs of nursing through care plans or workload measures; we have the equivalent of the doctor's Read Codes (Read, 1992) being developed for nursing; and we have nursing audit attempting to demonstrate nursing outcomes. All of these tackling different parts of the costs and benefits of nursing.

The Value for Money Equation (Figure 4.1) resulted from a desire to determine an integrated way of measuring the costs in relation to the benefits of nursing, while remaining patient focused. It treats the patient's requirements for nursing as a product line. In production terms there must be both inputs, and outputs.

Inputs

Inputs (in the case of the patient's requirements for nursing) are the costs of that nursing time and the competence or skills that the nurse has to meet those needs. In many instances, costs are used to equal skills as it is assumed that a higher paid (and therefore higher grade) nurse will have more skills. This ignores the variety of skills within grades, i.e. all E grade nurses do not have the exact same expertise or abilities. In fact, a Sister may select a new E grade nurse to complement the whole team's expertise, e.g. looking for an E grade who has a teaching and assessing qualification, another who has a counselling qualification, another who has intensive care experience, and another who has skills in therapeutic massage etc.

There are several ways to measure costs:

1. *Cost per day/diem* This is the average nursing cost per patient day, i.e. the total nursing cost of the service divided by the number of patient days.
2. *Cost per diagnosis method* This is the standard nursing care costs per patient diagnosis. For this method, a standard care profile is identified which incorporates the resources most commonly used and available. It is costed for average nurse costs per hour. This runs into difficulties when deciding an initial diagnosis. It also related to a medical model. While this is useful in ensuring consistency and compatibility with costing systems for medical inputs, it does not necessarily reflect the

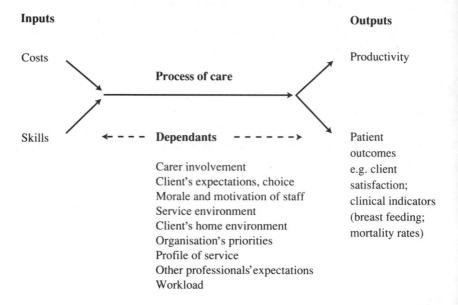

Figure 4.1 The value for money equation

nursing needs of the patient or tackle those patients whose primary requirement is for nursing.

3. *Cost per relative intensity measure* This was developed because of inadequacies in the previous method accurately to reflect differences in patient acuity. It calculated the time spent on nursing and non-nursing tasks for the entirety of the patient stay, dividing patients into homogeneous groups based on the use of the nursing resource. Length of stay was found to be the single best predictor of nursing time required. It is work that has been undertaken predominantly in acute units.

4. *Cost per nursing workload* This links costs to diagnosis or cost centres by classifying the patient into a dependency category for which there are determined nurse hours. These hours are costed using direct and indirect categories. The patients are aggregated in Diagnostic Related Groups (DRGs) along with their costed nurse hours which are then analyed to provide a cost per DRG. This is probably most popular in the USA, partly because it was used originally to roster staff. This method is patient-focused, can be related to a medical model and can be linked to available staffing. However, it is detailed and labour intensive in the initial stages.

Competence

The nurse's ability to deliver the care required, or even to determine the best route of care, is dependent on personal competence. Achieving levels of competence also requires resource investment in training and reflective practice. The competence the nurse brings to the patient's problem will affect cost in terms of an overhead for all patients in relation to staff development, and the pay scale awarded to ensure that the nurse is competent. Thus, a measure that costs the nurse's time and relates that to competence is required. Again, a nurse may be knowledgeable but incompetent. Thus, the measure needs to take into consideration the effectiveness of that nurse. Inputs in terms of nursing time costs and staff development costs should be linked to outputs to draw correlation between costs and competence.

Outputs

Outputs can be seen in terms of productivity of the nurses (number of patients cared for and discharged) and patient outcomes (the outcomes of the nursing care delivered).

Productivity

This is the activity of number of patients treated. In terms of community nursing it would be the numbers of patients admitted to and discharged from the nurse's caseload, the total number on the caseload and the length of time patients stay on the caseload. This is a measure of the nurse's efficiency and effectiveness in successfully meeting the patient's goals or requirements for his/her particular skills. It must not be judged in isolation from the other key output which is patient outcomes. There is no point taking people off the caseload to meet productivity requirements if their health suffers as a consequence.

Outcomes

In order for this to be meaningful, outcomes must relate to the target outcomes agreed between the patient and the nurse. As mentioned previously, patient motivation and priorities should influence goal setting in relation to outcome. Outcome can be measured by assessing the patient's perceived and actual problems using validated assessment criteria such as:

Functional mobility
Pain
Social adjustments

Psychological status
Health indices

Outcome can also be measured against known clinical indicators of care, e.g. pressure sore prevalence rate, incontinence levels, leg ulcer healing rates. Once assessed, the joint expectations in improving this assessment can be recorded and reassessed on discharge from the nurse's service. The difference in health status from admission to discharge, and any difference between expectations and actual achievement can then be used as a measure of patient outcome and as a tool for audit. This should be linked to patient satisfaction through interviews, as an outcome, thus combining health indicators with patient satisfaction. Finally, outputs should be compared to what can be expected from staff of the calibre employed. For instance, it may be the case that all nurses in the study use an outdated method of caring for leg ulcers, which prolongs healing. Only by auditing the nursing care against national good practice can we be sure that we are getting the optimum cost benefits framework.

Process

Looking at inputs and outputs provides a somewhat simplified picture of a patient's experience. There are other factors besides costs and skills that effect the overall outputs; these are the actual care process put in place (treatment package and care plan) and factors described in the model as 'dependants'. These dependent factors recognise the human world in which we live and our desire to provide a personalised service for empowered patients. Thus the professional's ability or willingness to achieve the desired outputs for a particular patient group will be determined by:

a) That professional's morale and motivation.
b) The involvement of the carers in providing care.
c) The individual patient's personal choice in care planning, and their expectations of the outcome.
d) The service environment.
e) The patient's home environment.
f) The organisation's priorities (purchaser and provider).
g) The professional team's total workload.

Morale and motivation   There is plenty of research that supports the theory that motivated and valued staff enjoy their work and produce a better service for patients. However skilled the nurse may be and however much he or she is paid, if his contribution is not valued his work will be of a lower standard.

Involvement of the carers in providing care   This can affect the overall workload of the nurse and the ability of the nurse to discharge the patient. If the carers are willing and involved they may take over the whole of the patient's care increasing the nurse's productivity. However, if the carers are unhappy with the overall outcome, they may refuse to take over the patient's care.

The individual patient's personal choice in care planning, and their expectations of the outcome   For example, the patient may present with a physical and an emotional problem. The doctor or nurse may perceive the former to be the most important and devote time and resources to that; the patient may perceive the latter to be the most important and feel let down by the care received. This brings in another dimension to costing, which is appropriateness. The question must be asked 'Did the care given solve the patient's problem?' Only the patient can reply. Moreover, the patient may choose not to comply with the recommendations of the nurse (e.g. to give up smoking prior to surgery), thus increasing the length of stay or contributing to a poor outcome.

The service environment   The environment in which the patient is being cared for (e.g. the quality of the mattress) will have an impact on the nurse's ability to prevent pressure sores and infections. Costs can be accentuated by the fact the nurse is running around trying to find a bed, rather than by competence inadequacies.

The patient's home environment   The ability to discharge a patient is dependent on home circumstances. Thus, the overlap between social, private and NHS care will affect both the inputs and the outputs.

The organisation's priorities (purchaser and provider)   If the organisation views one type of patient a lower priority, or chooses to channel resources towards other areas of its activities, this will impact on both inputs and outputs.

Workload   The needs of any one patient must be viewed in terms of the needs of all the patients on the caseload of the team and the ability of the team to meet those needs.

This value for money equation links information obtained from resource management (e.g. costs, productivity, care process, workload), quality (e.g. patient satisfaction) and audit (e.g. clinical outcomes, care process), while adding in information to complete the whole picture.

Conclusion

Trust status implies a corporate identity and culture which in turn suggests the pursuit of integrated audit and quality assurance, to achieve constant standards. With clearer corporate goals and philosophy, internal boundary problems between departments should diminish as everyone pursues the same corporate ends. (Harman and Martin, 1991)

Managers, be they clinical directors or service managers, require information on the dynamic of the patient's experience to enable them to make resource decisions. Purchasers require value for money within their contract. Patients/consumers expect the service to be developing better quality solutions to their problems and to enhance their total health care experience. Systems should be in place to ensure that current research informs current practice. Audit should thus form the development arm of research ensuring that research is implemented in practice.

Audit is now accepted in a multidisciplinary context, with some recognition that it will undoubtedly have a part to play in the contractual process (see Chapter 8). In addition, clinical staff (doctors, nurses and therapists) are beginning to define their information requirements, often with the benefits of the lessons learned from the RM initiative. These information requirements serve the purpose of caseload management, which includes clinical care decisions and management of the whole patient's experience. This blurring and softening of the edges of audit means that it is possible to explore the links between other major initiatives, namely resource management and quality. Moreover the instigation of the research and development strategy within the NHS clearly provides opportunities of linking research to audit, to the management of resources and decisions about service delivery. Many provider units are exploring the relationship between all these and are seeking to subsume audit under the umbrella (in the majority) of quality or (in the minority) of resource management (Figure 4.2). Thus, audit is becoming integral to the quality systems being developed and clinical information systems are replacing or being developed from existing RM information systems. Audit is seen as the opportunity to really pull clinical staff into the corporate workings of the Trust, even though this will take some considerable time to achieve. The danger, with the underlying current of desire to directly involve doctors in management decisions, is that the other professions, who must become equal partners in audit if change is to be meaningful, may yet again be marginalised, jeopardising the opportunity to achieve fundamental improvements in care.

The contracting process will not allow medical audit to remain a secretive activity in isolation from broader quality initiatives and from resource management. If clinicians and managers want to secure contracts, they will have to demonstrate continuous quality improvement within reasonable resources. In order to maximise the impetus of the seemingly separate initiatives of quality, resource management and audit, hospital and community units must seek to look for areas of commonality and develop an overall strategy that incorporates all facets of each initiative. In order to achieve this, organisations will need to view the client's total experience in the context of the value for money equation and the abilities of the health care professionals to meet client needs.

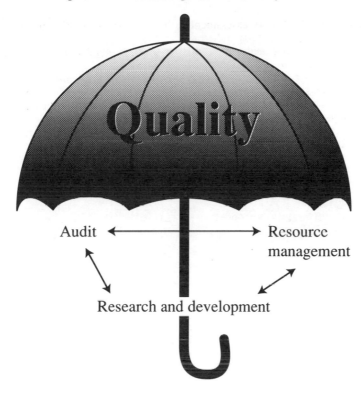

Audit ← → Resource management

Research and development

Figure 4.2 The umbrella of quality

References

Bagust A and Burrows J (1992) Quality or quantity. *Health Services Journal*, 6 August: 23–25.

Berwick D, Enthoven A, and Bunker J (1992) Quality management in the NHS: the doctor's role − 1. In R Smith (ed) *Audit in Action*. Plymouth: *British Medical Journal*.

Black N and Thompson E (1993) Obstacles to medical audit: British doctors speak. *Social Science and Medicine*, **36**, 7: 849–856.

Buchan J and Ball J (1991) *Caring Costs*. IMS Report No 208. Brighton: Institute of Manpower Studies.

Donabedian A (1990) The quality of care: how can it be assessed? In N O Graham (ed) *Quality Assurance in Hospitals: Strategies for Assessment and Implementation*. Rockville, Maryland: Aspen Publishers.

Edwardson S and Giovannetti P B (1987) A review of cost accounting methods for nursing services, *Nursing Economics*, **5**, 3: 107–117.

Harman D and Martin G (1991) *Medical Audit and the Manager*. Birmingham: Health Services Management Centre.

Kitson A (1989) *A Framework For Quality*. Royal College of Nursing Standards of Care Group. London: Royal College of Nursing.

Maxwell R J (1984) Quality assessment in health. *British Medical Journal*, **288**: 1470–1472.

Mosley J (1992) Using audit in a district-wide management system. *Health Services Management*, July/August: 27–29.

Packwood T, Keen J. and Buxton M (1991) *Hospitals in Transition*. Bristol: Open University Press.

Read J (1992) The Read Codes: repesenting the language of health care providers in computers. *Times Health Supplement*, July/August: 2–4.

Walshe K and Coles J (1993) *Evaluating Audit: Developing a Framework*. London: CASPE Research.

5

The Key to Audit in the Community

Caring for people – community care in the next decade and beyond

From the context of the White Paper issued by the Secretary of State stems the urgent need for the clarification of professional roles and responsibilities, the coordination of relevant sources of finance, and the identification of individuals at local level to take responsibility and be accountable for decision making. *Caring for people* is also the major launch pad for shifting the purchasing arrangements for health and social care in the community to local authorities who have assumed responsibility for buying residential services for both long- and short-term care, working collaboratively with health authorities in this aim.

The important fundamental objectives that underpin caring for people are at risk of being diluted because of the delays experienced in implementation of the act. Before care in the community can be evaluated by sound audit measures it is perhaps useful to rehearse the fundamental objectives as clarified by Smith (1993):

- To promote the development of domiciliary, day and respite services to enable people to live in their own homes wherever feasible.
- To ensure that service providers make practical support for carers a high priority.
- To make proper assessment of need and to make good case management the cornerstone of high quality care.
- To promote the development of a flourishing independent sector alongside good quality public services.
- To clarify the responsibilities of agencies and so make it easier to hold them to account for their performance.
- To secure value for taxpayers' money by introducing a new funding structure for social care.

With these objectives in mind, the successful implementation of community care is dependent wholly on good interorganisational relationships and all professionals working together. Health professionals are therefore supporting clients/patients (with more and more complex health or social problems) in their own homes or home-like settings. In these circumstances, health professionals will need to audit the outcome of the care packages in order to convince purchasers of the quality of service delivery. Health authorities are seen as providing health care and are expected to work collaboratively with social services by ensuring that health experts such as clinicians, community nurses and therapists take part in a needs assessment.

The main ethos of caring for people in the community is enabling those who are classified as vulnerable to be supported at home. However, assessment of need for this client group has its problems. If the social care needs are fragile, this may have an effect on the individual's health or mental health needs.

In order to develop effective care packages, there is a requirement for sound skills in networking across professional boundaries, advocacy, critical analysis and definition of the needs of clients and carers. Assessment tools can be tailored to accommodate the special requirements of client groups being served.

Within this new culture, the Community Care Acts asks care managers to be conversant with criteria for client entry to individual services. The natural continuum for this is the development of periodic assessment for individual services to demonstrate outcomes as part of the audit cycle; this would need to bridge local authority and health authority services. Part of this bridge is the joint appointment of a care manager, working as an integral part of the primary healthcare team. As work has developed in the formulation of criteria for referral of care management and the production of comprehensive and realistic joint assessment tools, the gate has been opened wide for the development of primary healthcare audit tools.

The care manager's role is the lynch pin for introducing collaborative audit measures; much work will have to be done in marketing this role and gaining an understanding within primary health care teams of its overlapping remit in relation to social services, district nursing services and community psychiatric nursing services, for example.

The care manager is responsible for co-ordinating the production of a dynamic assessment and audit tool and is best placed for this role as he or she is independent from the provision of services. The care manager also brings a different perspective to the audit process, that of the purchasing perspective in a micro-commissioning role.

Central to the reforms, the care manager will be coordinating an integrated assessment and referral system. There is now considerable experience across the country of care managers using a single assessment which is multi-faceted, specifically for each health service discipline involved. There is, however, some conflict in the care manager's role which must be guarded against. This arises where the role combines being an assessor of needs as well as a budget holder for provision. The realistic needs of patients and carers may be compromised as described by Morris (1993):

> If care managers are assessors and budget holders, the incentive to restrict assessment to what can be provided will rest with one person . . . Needs-led assessment may turn out to be nothing more than a disguise for resource-led assessment.

This does need to be balanced with the knowledge that there are clear criteria for accepting and making onward appropriate referrals. The individual care package, which is tailored to patient/carer need, must be clear and precise as to the services offered and the outcome expected.

Jackson (1993) suggests that the key to the implementation of these reforms is the efficacy of care management and the growth and experience of care managers in assessing clients needs, developing appropriate care packages and monitoring their implementation, all of which will need careful auditing.

Care management

The success of using care management to increase the efficient use of community based services for the long-term care of elderly people with physical or learning disabilities or people with mental illness will need to be evaluated. From within care management grows the new role of the care manager as previously described. Most have been trained and worked as community nurses, social workers, home care organisers or other professionals. Grove (1992) highlights the fact that care managers could be seen as roughly the social service equivalent of fundholding general practitioners. She goes on to point out that unlike GPs, care managers will not actually deliver care themselves, rather they will organise multidisciplinary assessments for people needing help and will then try to arrange exactly what is needed.

Parker *et al* (1990) suggest a definition for case management as follows:

> A systematic process of assessment, planning, service co-ordination and/or referral, and monitoring and reassessment through which the service needs of clients are met.

Griffiths (1989) has described case management as 'the cornerstone to community care'; it is an approach which identifies people's needs and links this into a method of ensuring that clients' changing needs are continually reviewed, based on regular assessments of the care needs of individuals and their carers. Existing referral systems should be evaluated regularly and all care packages should be based on clearly defined objectives which ensure that delivery of care is secured through regular monitoring of the quality and outcome of care.

The framework described by Griffiths lends itself particularly well to the implementation of caring for people by setting up an environment which will enable audit to flourish, for example, linking the processes of critical pathways, managed care and case management. Research is now required to establish the impact of care management in preventative services, the effect on health outcomes and cost effectiveness.

Care profiles

To enable appropriate care profiles to be developed, they need to be based on certain groupings or categories identified by diagnosis, by their high cost or by general practitioners. For each category, a draft format for a care profile can be drawn up to indicate, in timed sequences, the pattern of events of a selected management route for an episode of patient care (as shown in Figure 5.1).

Critical paths

This is a method by which key events are identified and depicted as a critical path, achieved by plotting the best possible patient outcome within planned resources and activities for selected patient types. The key objectives are to standardise outcomes and cost of care, while ensuring the best mix of resources and methods to achieve clinical and patient outcomes. Importantly, this method helps minimise duplication and variation in the clinical management process, and also helps to promote collaborative practice between health and social services. The key benefits are firstly that it helps patients develop a better understanding of those things in their treatment which have impacted positively on the outcome and it also produces professional satisfaction for staff, by linking their activities to identifiable patient outcomes. The best format for establishing critical paths within community or primary care should be based on a multi-disciplinary approach as this helps to ensure that joint working is truly taking place.

Managed care

The coordination of care is the focus of managed care, using the critical pathways to monitor such things as outcomes of care for individual patient case types and use of resources. It provides a framework for collaboration

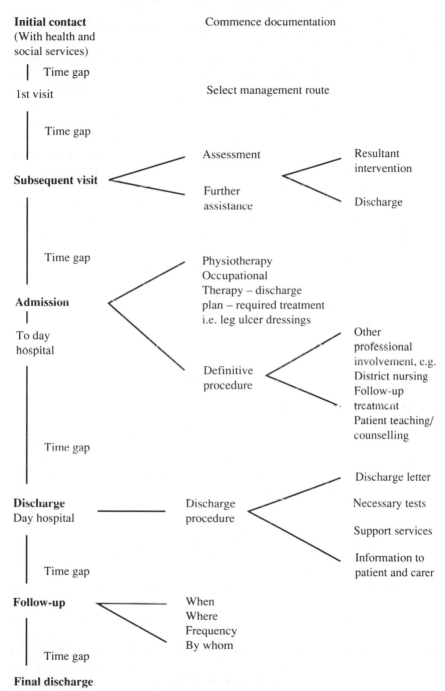

Figure 5.1 Sample care profile – failure to cope

in which clinical care is organised in sequence. This model of patient care has many benefits, such as providing continuity, linking tasks, duty rotas and different parts of the organisation (i.e. health centre). Case management, as previously discussed, provides a continuity by linking the care given across different clinical settings. The three frameworks for care identified above not only provide a sound platform for the foundations of clinical audit to be established but also enable audit to be built into the work of individual practitioners and primary health care teams.

A quality assurance strategy for both community and primary health care should reflect success in preventing and resolving health problems, to discover what is happening in a given patient episode and to amend or improve this experience in the future. There should be standards against which to measure care, to spread good practices and to monitor adverse patient occurrences; this should be achieved by identifying the application of external and internal clinical audits and performance-based criteria.

Contribution to community health care planning

The Black Report (1980) first identified the health gap between the affluent and the poor and this was more recently corroborated by a report by the Association of Community Health Councils, England and Wales (ACHCEW). This report identified that the health gap is continuing to widen and that a disproportionate number of deaths from tuberculosis, hypertension, violence and accidents occur among ethnic minorities. In the context of community care planning, there appears to be little doubt about the magnitude and complexity of this problem and it is therefore important that primary health care teams focus on a local assessment of community care, encompassing audit tools which will help to evaluate the following:

- Development of a profile of the practice locality.
- Identification of potential and actual patient needs in the practice population.
- Analysis of workload and caseload in the light of appropriate skill mix and expertise within the primary health care team.
- An assessment of what patients and carers experienced of the services offered.
- The practice profile should show such things as patterns and trends in morbidity and mortality, social and environmental characteristics and demographic trends and information of the effects of class, gender and race, as well as the impact of the sociology of health and illness of the population.

Creating a climate for audit in the community

Before audit can be successfully implemented in primary health care and within the community, it is important that a beneficial climate for audit is established. It is natural and understandable that people should feel initially resistant to being involved; this could be attributed to some of the definitions, such as 'audit is a calling to account'. This has many negative connotations and people may feel threatened by it.

In order to help facilitate the climate for audit there is a need to assess the work climate as perceived by each staff member. This can be done by using a confidential survey which would be sent to all field staff, managers and educators. The major focus of this tool would be to identify satisfaction related to communication within all levels of management, their perceptions of the work environment, whether they feel valued and empowered, and their frustrations. The results of this survey should be shared widely with all staff and action groups should be set up to work on both the positive and negative results, e.g. if communications are a problem one group needs to formulate a communication strategy which will be owned by the workforce and, therefore, fully implemented.

Resistance to audit or any major change manifests itself in many different ways. The apparent disinterest in audit is often because people feel threatened and anxious that audit will put them continually in the 'spotlight' and they may view it as a management stick to discipline them. In order to establish a positive climate for audit, it should be thought of in terms of systematic review of practice, identification of problems, development of possible solutions, implementation of change and further review. It depends on the motivation of committed clinically based staff to succeed. Creating an environment for this to happen must include a bottom up approach which encourages staff to identify priorities and goals in the knowledge that significant and valid changes can be made. Much of the audit culture needed to motivate change must be grown not only from the availability of resources, reliability and validity of data collecting methods but should rely heavily on the commitment of participants. In describing such an approach, Morison (1992) says 'the bottom up approach fosters a critical, questioning approach in nurses to their activities and encourages the notion of individual, professional accountability'.

Planning for change should take place before successful audit can be introduced, Green (1993) says that in order to introduce a planned change process, there is a need for a conscious, deliberate, collaborative effort to improve the operation of a system via the application of scientific knowledge. It involves mutual goal setting and the use of a change agent. Therefore, in order to establish the baseline for the introduction of audit, a pre-change evaluation will need to be carried out with the following data collected from staff:

- What is understood about audit, what is currently being audited and in what way?
- How would staff want to pursue audit further?
- Is there a place for a review of current service provision? Lewin (1951) suggests that the 'unfreezing' phase of the process where the organisation or the group recognises the need for change, identifies problems and attempts to resolve them. This unfreezing phase should then be backed up by raising awareness of the need for audit. Plant (1987) suggests that another important activity ensuring successful change involves mobilising energy and commitment to change.
- Is there a good peer review system? Within the process of culture change there needs to be a focus on establishing a good peer review system which is viewed as one element of a professional practice climate related to community and primary healthcare, evaluation of patient outcomes, quality assurance and self-governance. The purpose of the peer review system should be to evaluate professional practice of individuals or groups in relation to established standards with the aim of providing evidence to improve professional practice of the individual or group.
- A positive climate for enquiry is important from the outset and audit should be seen as an important component of continuing professional practice.

Designing and implementing a strategy for nursing and therapy audit

In these times of consumer participation, cost containment and market principles in the NHS, it is imperative that before rationing healthcare, decisions about service delivery are made. These decisions should be based on reliable methods of assessing and auditing both the quality and quantity of what is provided. In order to do this, provider performance must be assessed using outcomes in the context of the particular situation in which care takes place. Measuring tools should also encompass mechanisms of measurement the achievement of stated goals, individual or team performance, problem identification and quality control.

Collaborative working

Over the last few years, many of the professions have been working on defining and re-defining specific audit tools to measure outcomes of their practice. Much of the experience in this work has been carried out in acute settings practising uniprofessional audit. Only latterly has there been a move to bring together this experience and expertise, tailoring it and refining it into the beginnings of collaborative audit. The community, however, is more complex and the growth of audit in this environment has been slightly restrained due to the fact that primary care is somewhat different from hospital care. For instance, in the acute setting, the admission and discharge have set defined parameters for audit to take place. The identification of when an illness starts and when it ends can be difficult in the community. Christoffel and Lowenthall (1977) say that 'There is difficulty developing a uniform system for quality assurance in the community since the settings in primary care vary considerably. These may be in the patients' homes, in the surgery, in a department within the health centre.' The authors also suggest that it is easier to audit within a hospital setting where the patient is part of a captive audience, as opposed to primary care where it is up to the patients themselves to decide whether they come for follow-ups or repeat visits to the health centre. Another possible reason why audit has not taken off quite so quickly in the community is that, within uniprofesional audit, some of the methods professionals use to collect information are not as structured as those used within an acute setting. For instance, Littlewood (1985) suggested that district nurses were often overworked and the job understaffed, which had a particular effect on such things as the use of the nursing process. It was found that a very low percentage of district nurses recorded or used the evaluation section. If this is the case, then one of the important foundations for audit is absent.

For audit to be an effective way of measuring outcomes of any care intervention within the health and social care interface, the infrastructure for this to happen must be worked at and established in parallel to developing audit measures and tools. In order to achieve this objective the use of the **key model** can be of great assistance to set markers for the infrastructure and to ensure that all the activities within it are worked concurrently alongside audit. Thus, all activities are completely integrated and interactive, ensuring that no one activity is carried out independently. The key model can be used as a uniprofessional framework or a collaborative framework.

The key model

To establish the evolution and state of audit in the community, the nursing profession is used to illustrate the experience of implementing audit in this setting. The key model for quality assurance is used in this example as a model to unlock the door to nursing audit within a district nursing service. The key model encompasses eight characteristics which will need to be run concurrently. The framework that underpins this model is as follows:

i)   It provides a planned systematic approach.
ii)   It is a bottom-up approach to quality assurance.
iii)   It provides a combination of data retrieval methods.
iv)   It is integrated into all nursing functions.
v)   It is strongly integrated with nursing standards.

The eight activities of the key model provide the structure around the mechanisms needed to operate, direct and control the nursing service, as shown in Figure 5.2. These eight key components formed the basis of a major review of a district nursing service in the south of England. In order to respect the rapid changes that were occurring within the National Health Service when this review started, the service needed to be structured to enable it not only to be well informed about the specific content of clinical roles but also to be knowledgeable regarding the social pressures, forces and processes that influenced the changes in the role of nursing. District nurses needed to look at the environment in which change occurred in terms of the forces that facilitated as well as those that impeded change.

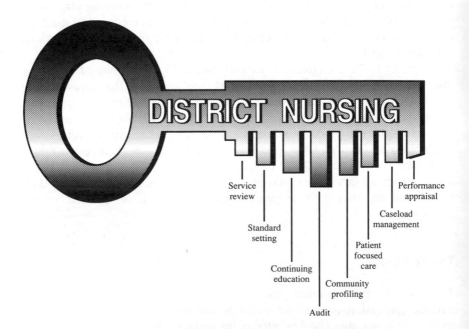

Figure 5.2 The key model

Service review

> - Successful implementation of 'caring for people' depends on skills in networking across professional boundaries, advocacy, critical analysis and sound assessment skills
> - Central to the reforms is the new role of 'care manager'
> - Development of dynamic assessment and audit tools
> - Profiling of skill mix

Although the district nursing service was highly rated by the community at large, district nurses felt that, in order to address the new health agenda for the 1990s, they needed to move the service forward from being one that was essentially illness dominated to one that had a clear idea of long-term health goals as they related to local needs. The service was split into four geographical patches which were not coterminous with social services. The four patches had their own night nursing service which meant that they were often rather insular, with no corporate objectives and no overall long-term planning over such issues as:

i)   *Staffing* Cover was not provided for sickness, holidays, etc. from other patches, resulting in a high reliance on bank staff.

ii) *Continuing education* No overall strategy was followed for the whole service, for example, educational needs were identified by nurses' own personal preference.

iii) *Health needs of the population* These were not being met by the nursing service and initiatives such as well women clinics and diabetic clinics were more of a reflection of practitioner interest rather than a clear identification of need.

iv) *Skill mix* Within the patches, skill mix had been determined more by custom and practice then by enquiry into workload.

In early 1990 a series of workshops were established for district nurses and these centred around the following themes:

i)   To consider the impact of current government health care initiatives.

ii) To determine the needs of Project 2000 students/nurses in the community.

iii) To begin to identify different patterns of skill mix by reviewing existing structures.

iv) To become aware of cost effective, cost–benefit issues.

v)   To have a commitment to active caseload management.

vi) To consider strategies for change to address future health care needs in the community within existing resources.

From these workshops a four-day district nursing development programme emerged, the format of which is shown below:

District Nursing Development Programme
Day 1
Organisational culture
The climate of change to include conflict issues

Day 2
Introduction to primary nursing
Comparison of current and proposed nursing practice
Role clarification
Personal development

Day 3
Legal and ethical issues
Accountability
Safe practice
Maintaining professional issues

Day 4
The process of audit, including standard settings
Monitoring outcomes
Audit results
The need for research
The change environment

All members of the district nursing service attended this programme, the
main themes of which were evaluated so that feedback could be incorporated positively into service plans and contracts. This enabled the workforce to feel valued and to have some degree of control of the direction in
which the service was moving.

Resulting from the workshops, the district nursing service had to be
restructured in a way that produced a new breed of managers. Firstly, an
assistant nurse manager post was established with responsibility for setting
up research projects to underpin clinical practice outcomes and with

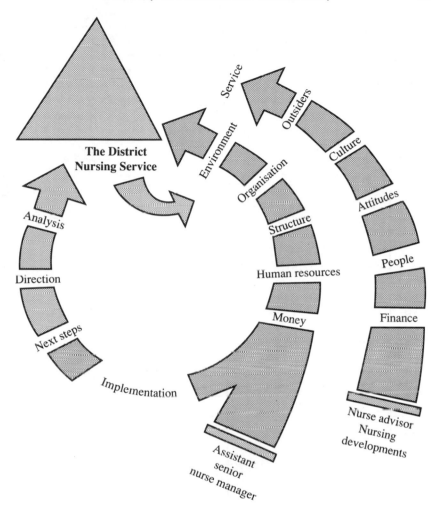

Figure 5.3 A review of a district nursing service

managerial responsibility for three nursing teams to ensure a more corporate overall management style. Secondly, a nurse adviser (nursing developments) was appointed to act as an agent of change within the service to raise standards of clinical care (Figure 5.3). The nursing workforce was established into three teams led by a clinical nurse manager; these teams were coterminous with social services patches as shown in Figure 5.4.

The district nurse as a nurse practitioner

As part of the service review, nursing staff felt that it was important to examine the nurse practitioner role and extrapolate the pivotal functions

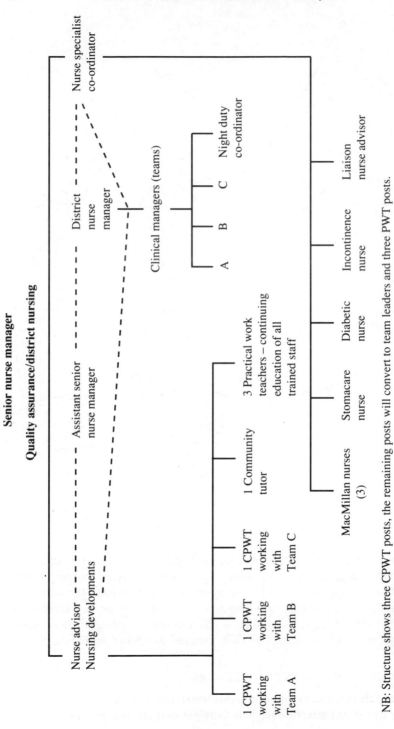

Figure 5.4 Proposed new structure for the district nursing service senior nurse manager quality assurance/district nursing

that underpin it. In order to obtain a clear definition of a nurse practitioner it was thought helpful to examine both the clinical nurse specialist and the nurse practitioner as this helped to identify where and how these roles were sometimes blurred, causing a lack of understanding of both roles in the past.

Clinical nurse specialist

The clinical nurse specialist or CNS role could be said to be a specialist nurse who provides highly focused nursing care for a defined caseload of patients in a given speciality. The CNS provides social and psychological support to patients, teaches patients and their families how to handle illness-related problems and serves as a resource and role model to other members of the health care team. These roles were often derived from a medical model based on diagnosis, such as diabetes, stomacare or asthma care.

The role of the nurse practitioner has been described as working collaboratively to manage holistically such things as chronic illnesses, to provide health advice to mothers and children, to empower patients by informing them on all aspects of health care and to treat minor acute illnesses and injuries. This new knowledge base is drawn primarily from medicine but the role gave nurses better opportunities to provide flexible nursing care packages which often incorporated competencies derived from medicine and other paramedical professionals. Many of these roles were pioneering in origin, working with the homeless and unregistered patients. The role of the nurse practitioner is often confused and has in the past been described as a support role to medicine, being expressed in terms of tasks the nurse can perform.

As work progressed on the service review it seemed that the clinical nurse specialist role identified closely with the advanced practitioner role and that the time had come for staff to take stock of the nurse practitioner role, the models for which have, in many instances, been imported from Canada and the USA and are often mismatched with our health service, health needs and culture. It was felt that the time had come for a new vision which should help, support and prepare nurses to work towards the goal of becoming independent or autonomous practitioners, advancing their nursing practice in a generic way but focusing on the requirements of special client groups or needs.

The new UKCC Code of Conduct *The Scope of Professional Practice* (1992) for the first time gives nurses the opportunity to develop roles which are not medically driven but needs driven and patient focused, derived from the values of nursing.

Nurses felt that the autonomous practitioner role should provide an open access service to patients and their families and allows the nurse's role to expand and extend to address gaps in the health care delivery system, and allows nurses to gain recognition as high quality, cost-effective providers. It was decided that these new roles should be based on the following criteria:

Empowerment of patients   The ability to support, inform and guide patients to make informed decisions about their own health care. The ability to help patients to make choices and have ownership and control of their own care packages.

Patient-focused care   The service must:

- Be patient-focused.
- Improve quality of care for patients.
- Satisfy patients and staff.
- Be easily accessible for patients and relatives, i.e. operate open access.

Therapeutic practice

- The process for achieving best nursing practice should be strategically planned.
- That strategy should centre on empowering the patient.
- It requires a multitude of approaches.
- All approaches should incorporate the dissemination of practices which have been tried, tested and evaluated as successful.
- Development in practice should incorporate interagency and multidisciplinary collaboration.

  Achievement of best practice is not a competitive process but is dependent on networking. (*Achieving Best Nursing Practice*, Yorkshire RHA, 1992)

Collaborative work   Developments in practice should incorporate interagency and multidisciplinary collaboration. The roles should be grounded by a higher nursing degree and include the ability to teach, be a leader/manager, change agent, researcher and evaluator and investigator of nursing research.

- The role dimensions require the nurse practitioner to provide input, practice, education, consultation and research.
- Administering and monitoring therapeutic interventions and regimes.
- Effective management of rapidly changing situations.
- The diagnostic and monitoring function.
- Teaching/coaching function.
- Monitoring and ensuring the quality of health care practice.
- Organisational work and role competencies.

Advanced nursing skill base   Nurse practitioners should be masters prepared not only in the technical/medical tasks but, most importantly, in areas which are firmly grounded in nursing theory and practice:

- All advanced practice based on nursing research.
- All nurse practitioner roles should provide a skill base in health promotion and health and health maintenance activities.
- The advanced clinical abilities to provide primary health care to a variety of populations in different settings.
- All characteristics of a masters prepared nurse including the ability to be a teacher, leader/manager, change agent, researcher, evaluator and utiliser of nursing research.

Research-based practice   All nursing practice should be firmly grounded by research. However, for this to happen, there needs to be more commitment from nurse managers and general managers in resource terms.

Change agent role   The roles should be seen as internal agents of change whose focus is to innovate improve, advance and bridge all the nursing care practices in the community and hospital services.

Cost-effective care   This must be based on the measurements of outputs; variations in level of quality of care provided should be demonstrated by clear cost–benefit analysis.

A philosophy for district nursing

A philosophy of care which described the service in total was generated; it focused on providing professional skilled nursing care which was adapted to individual need within the home environment. Having developed a philosophy of care, the service then moved on to identify criteria for admission to the service as this would assist users to understand agreed criteria for referral of skilled nursing care. This was based on the following:

i)   Care and support which could be given by a family member or carer.
ii) Nursing care delivered by a nurse through empowering and supporting the family or carer to perform semi-skilled nursing functions.
iii) Skilled nursing care which can only be delivered by the district nursing team.

Following on from the philosophy and criteria for admission, there was an urgent need for some work to be done on role definition to ensure that there was appropriate use of skilled staff both to provide an efficient and effective service and to enhance job satisfaction. Each role within the team was profiled by skills analysis; teams were then matched in this way to provide nursing care for the health needs of the particular geographical patch.

Committee structure for district nursing service

It was felt that the committee structure for district nursing should form an important part of the organisation of the service in order to provide a more efficient flexible and fully informed team of nurses. A structure was designed to provide a district nursing executive, nursing policy committee, nursing practice/research committee and journal club (Figure 5.5).

Standard setting

- Definition of philosophy of care in community
- Identification of a values bank
- Development of standards of care which form a benchmark of good collaborative care
- Standards of care can then be audited to demonstrate outcome of collaborative care

A range of standards was set which had clearly defined outcomes; these covered areas such as evaluation of planned nursing care, pain management, individualised care, domiciliary nursing assessment and accessibility of the district nursing service.

Continuing education

- Shared learning strategies
- Peer group learning
- Professional practice (e.g. professional accreditation to demonstrate clinical competence)
- Educational/practical profiling of team members

The establishment of a team of three practical work teachers to work with trained district nurses and three to work with students enabled all nurses to have practical help to introduce change into the service. The postholders ensured that all trained staff were able to follow agreed practical training programmes to equip them for the provision of more acute nursing in the community. These posts are also of value in the transition to Project 2000 in the community setting. Much time was committed to identifying the training needs for the establishment of nurse practitioner roles for all trained district nurses. Before these could be identified all the specialist nursing roles required scrutiny.

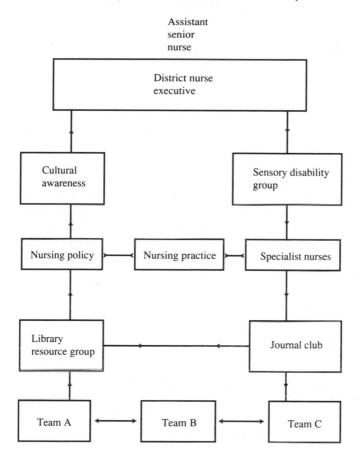

Figure 5.5 Committee structure for District Nursing Services

Audit

Nursing audit is part of the cycle of quality assurance. It incorporates the systematic and critical analyses by nurses, midwives and health visitors, in conjunction with other planning, delivery and evaluation of nursing and midwifery care, in terms of their use of resources and the outcomes for patients/clients, and introduces appropriate change in response to that analysis. (Project 32 NHS ME, 1991)

It was important for the service to define audit and explore the audit process and its relationship to standard setting initiatives that were already underway. A nursing audit sub-group was set up to establish a framework for audit and develop an audit tool. The group based their work on Shaw's framework for introducing quality assurance (1986) in which he identifies the following themes:

Appropriateness
Effectiveness
Acceptability
Continuity
Accessibility
Efficiency

Following this the nursing audit group adopted an outcomes perspective to enable a long-term commitment and adoption of an evaluative audit approach including careful measurements of inputs and activities. Outcome criteria were chosen based on a nursing diagnosis. Some were based on more of a medical model because they reflected a large proportion of the patient population, for example, rheumatology, diabetes mellitus and chronic airways disease. The audit outcome tool which was eventually designed required other work to be completed in parallel, such as, the development of standardised care plans and measurement tools to identify baselines with patients before nursing intervention took place, and responding post-nursing intervention assessment to demonstrate a response or change in the patient.

Workload targets and community profiling

> The individual district nurse practitioner takes continuous responsibility for:
> ● Assessment of health needs
> ● Planning of care package
> ● Implementation of care
> ● Evaluation of care given
> ● Reassessment of health needs

In order for caseload management to be effective:

● Regularly sample caseloads.
● *Process* Involve staff at all times in setting workload targets, monitor workload targets monthly, refine targets and make changes.
● *Evaluation* to determine: if health needs are met and outcomes achieved; effective management of human and financial resources; efficient information systems.

It was felt important that the service set broad workload targets which linked closely to the district health authority's corporate objectives. It was important that these workload targets should be identified both by field staff and their managers together. This required facilitation by an experienced nurse with research and community experience who was not employed in the service and could therefore bring some objectivity to the exercise. It was important to get over the concept that if staff time is being managed efficiently this has a direct bearing on the amount of nurse–patient contact time. Therefore, the broad targets that were set in the first year focused on:

(1) Increasing nurse–patient contact time.
(2) Rationalisation of travelling, e.g. re-zoning visits to reduce nurses' journey times.
(3) All domiciliary visits that on evaluation could not guarantee or demonstrate a clear gain in outcome to the patient were eliminated from caseloads.
(4) The more efficient and effective use of trained district nurses, e.g. the disbanding of a night nursing service and the establishment of an 'on call' night service, in order to increase service provision at other times of the day.

Success in meeting the above workload targets is shown in Figure 5.6.

The evaluation of these workload targets across all geographical patches required local assessment of the service delivered, the ability to meet health care needs, outcomes and efficient use of resources. It is encouraging to note that at an early stage, this work improved the management of resources within the district nursing service and regular audit of users' views demonstrated increased satisfaction.

The district nursing service served a resident population of 215,570 which was unlikely to change over the next decade. The district was a multicultural area with a significant ethnic minority which was predicted to rise to 24 per cent in the next decade. In 1981, the Borough had England's eleventh highest percentage of people whose head of household was born in the new Commonwealth of Pakistan; it had the largest Pakistani population in London. It is also suggested that the numbers over 65 years of age would increase from approximately 1 000 in 1981 to almost 4 000 in the

	1989/90 Service provision
Support services	Reduced by 5%
Travel	Reduced by 3%
Patient contact	Increased by 4%
Clinics (GP/Health centres)	Increased by 6%

Figure 5.6 Workload targets

cent of Borough's 65-plus population. With this in mind it was important for the district nursing service to establish a community profile. The format used was designed by Yorkshire Regional Health Authority in the following way:

A community will be defined in terms of a geographical neighbourhood or location or general practice population.

i) *Demographic data* Profile of population, at-risk groups, social class etc.
ii) *Geographical description of the area* Urban, rural, industrial, etc.
iii) *Description of service organisation* District nursing, locality, practice-based, etc.
iv) *Indicators of need*
  a. Market research.
  b. Epidemiological criteria – levels of ill health, morbidity/mortality rates etc.
  c. Particular factors that may create needs – hostels, caravan sites, drug abuse, etc.
  d. Office of Population Surveys (OPS) census measurements.
  e. Hospital waiting lists and discharge policy.
  f. Use of known tools of assessment – Jarman score.
v) *Resources available*
  a. District nurses, specialist nurses.
  b. Other staff available.
  c. Health authority owned facilities, health centres, day hospitals, etc.
  d. Other facilities – GP practices, social services, day centres, hospices etc.
  e. Community networks – local, voluntary provision.
  f. Use of known statistics – Fip, Korner.
  g. General issues that influence staffing – learner placements, staff developments etc.
  h. General issues that may effect the community – norms, values and traditions.

Patient-focused care

- Empowerment of small teams of district nurses
- Maximising the time that district spends on direct care giving
- Ensuring all nurses can see the direct impact of their care on patients
- Decreasing the number of district nurses who handle patient information

---

- Decreasing the distance district nurses patients and carers have to travel within health centres
- The introduction of a total quality management system that engenders exception reporting
- Clinical nursing protocols for all admissions to the service
- Concentration of nursing expertise with small teams of district nurses
- Commitment to the personal development of all staff
- Leadership of nursing through matrix management

In order to ensure that the district nursing service was a needs-led service and not based on professional intuition, convenience, prejudice and custom practice, a patient-focused model was felt to be an important philosophy for the service to adopt. The principles of patient-focused care were identified as follows by a sub-group of district nurses. The service must:

- Be patient-focused.
- Improve quality of care for patients.
- Satisfy patients and staff.
- Have clear lines of management.

Having identified the principles, the group went on to determine the process of patient-focused care.

- The empowerment of small teams of district nurses.
- Maximising the time that district nurses spend on direct care giving.
- Ensuring all district nursing staff can see the direct impact of the service on their patients.
- Decreasing the number of team members who handle patient information.
- Decreasing the geographical distance district nurses have to travel within geographical or practice populations.
- Introducing a total quality management system dependent upon exception reporting.
- Devising nursing protocols for all admissions and discharges to and from the service and implementing regular review systems for long-stay patients.
- Concentrating district nursing expertise (clinical).
- Ensuring commitment to personal development.
- Ensuring leadership of nursing through shared management.

With the criteria for patient-focused care as a framework, the district nursing service was able to establish a nursing development unit which heightened the services ability for critical thinking and increased the understanding and the extent to which they were accountable. The nursing development environment heightened the relationship responsibility between nurses and patients and helped nurses to understand that their responsibilities were more patient directed since the patient was viewed as the centre of the organisation.

Caseload management

Checklist for caseload management
- Assessment of health needs
- Planning of care package
- Implementation of care
- Evaluation of care given
- Reassessment of health needs

In order for caseload management to take place effectively:

- Regularly sample caseloads.
- Identify categories of patients recently referred to the service.
- Identify patient categories who 'stay' on the books.
- Identify patients discharged from the service.
- Check that nurses' caseloads are reflective of local community in terms of sex, age or ethnic origin.
- Audit GP referral patterns.

The individual district nurse practitioner takes continual responsibility for assessment, planning, implementation and evaluation of health needs and the nursing care for patients' families and carers in the community. The autonomy of caseload management which is a prerequisite for this role includes the admission, discharge and transfer of patients from the service; this is an important, if not unique, responsibility vested in the district nurse. Therefore, it is seen as imperative that nurses develop competence in prioritising workloads and in the efficient use of personal and material resources.

In order for district nurse caseload management to take place, a sample review of the caseloads of all nursing teams was completed. This replicated the work carried out by Badger *et al* (1989) in central Birmingham which identified that recently referred patients were either terminally ill or had more chronic physical disorders. Patients who stayed on the books received either injections or general care from qualified staff or bathroom nursing auxiliaries; as in Badger's work there was also some concern that nurses' caseloads were not reflective of the local community in terms of sex, age or ethnic origin. An element of this may be due to the referral patterns from General Practitioners who perhaps do not refer certain categories of patients (Evers *et al*, 1988).

It was felt that a strategy for caseload management needed to incorporate frequent reassessment of patients on individual caseloads and analysis of referrals, length of stay and discharge from the service. In order to progress caseload management within the district nursing service, the following basic categories were used to analyse district nurse caseloads:

i)   Insulin daily or twice a day (no other injections included).
ii)   General nursing care (GNC), which may include washing, dressing, surgical dressing, bowel care, special procedures (e.g. tracheostomy care).
iii)   Dressings of various frequency.
iv)   Supervisory visits (SV) to patients needing advice and support rather than nursing care. This group includes terminal patients and those who have received more intensive care in the past and are now being monitored.
v)   Bath/wash (B/W). Patients who are part of the caseload because they need help with personal hygiene. The patients are usually visited weekly or fortnightly.
vi)   Injections (excluding insulin). Almost without exception these patients are visited either monthly or bi-monthly and in some cases three monthly for neo-cytamen injections.
vii)   Others   includes visits to patients needing oral medication either daily or to fill tablet dispensers, eye drops, catheter care, blood pressure checks and blood glucose monitoring.

Following identification of the above categorisation of nursing functions regular caseload analysis was carried out on a monthly basis, scrutinising all caseloads in the three geographic areas. For example, the contents of 10 caseloads were looked at in Area A with the numbers of caseloads varying from 18 patients to 35 (Figure 5.7). The analysis was carried out by looking at the numbers of visits taken to implement the care. The implementation varied considerably, ranging from 86 visits to 267 (Figure 5.8).

Caseload analysis health centre based for Team 'C'

Caseload numbers at Team C base vary between 11 patients (caseload of a part-time sister) to 40 patients (Figure 5.9). Some interesting points have been raised which differ from other areas that have been analysed.

1. Although the caseload numbers vary considerably, when looking at the number of visits required to implement them there is not such a wide variation in the number of visits required per month, apart from caseload 2 (Figure 5.10). It is interesting to note that caseload 4, with only 17 patients, needs 300 visits a month to implement the care plan and yet caseload 3 with 40 patients only needs 314 visits.

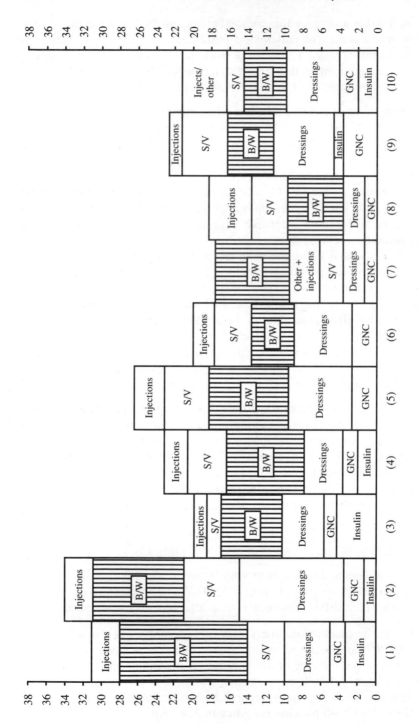

Figure 5.7 Caseloads of district nurses in Team 'A'
(*by number and type of patient on caseload, which is health centre based*)

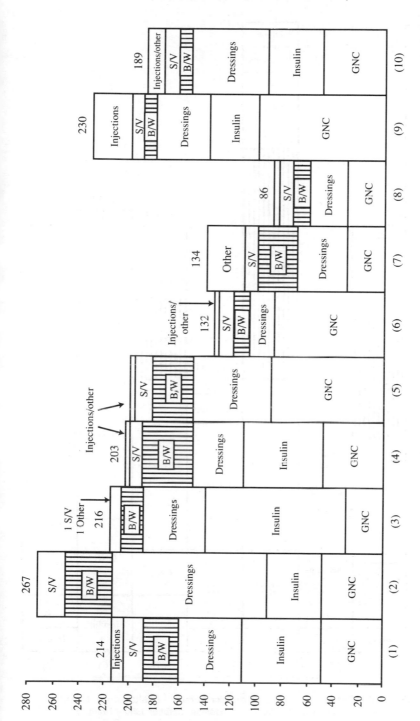

Figure 5.8 Graph showing number of visits required per caseload in Team 'A' (by number and type of visit for care plans to be implemented over a 4-week period)

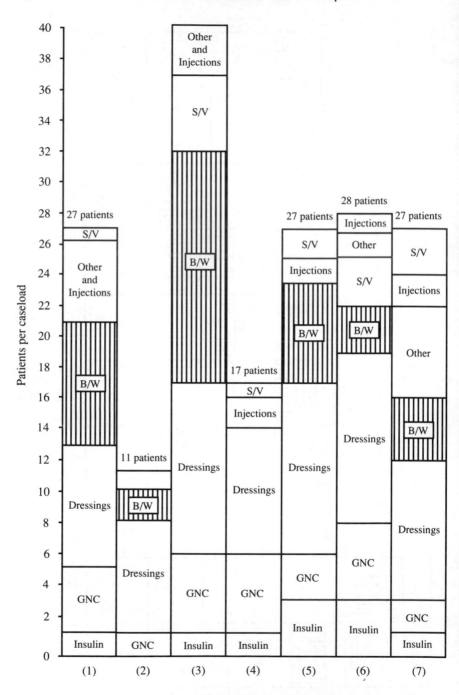

Figure 5.9 Caseload analysis of district nurses – health centre based
(by number and type of patients on caseload, October 1990 – Team C)

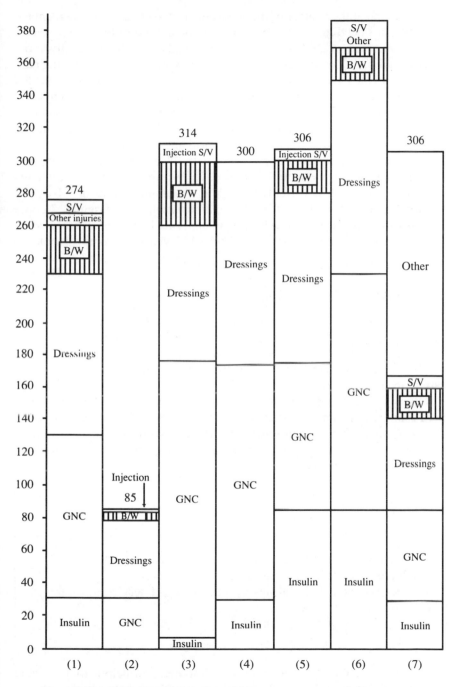

Figure 5.10 Visits required to implement care plan over a 28-day period
(Health centre based – Team C by number and type of visit)

Looking at the content of these caseloads, No. 3 has a high percentage of patients needing general nursing care on a daily or twice daily basis, most of which would be time consuming visits. Looking generally at the caseloads, a higher percentage of time is devoted to general nursing care (GNC) in the caseloads at Team C base than in other areas. This has led to the historic feeling that Team C base has a very heavy workload.

2. It is interesting to note that in Team C far fewer visits are categorised as 'bath/strip wash' than in other areas – possibly due to the pressure of work in the past and the need for prioritising of caseloads.

3. To compare caseloads 5 and 7, both with 27 patients and needing 306 visits per month, the actual time needed to implement those caseloads varies considerably. Caseload 5 has a higher proportion of GNC, but more importantly 142 of the 306 visits to implement caseload 7 come under the category 'other' which is an abnormally high percentage when comparing with other caseloads. These 142 visits are composed of:

(i)   One twice daily eye drops (56 visits)
(ii)   Three daily (oral) medications (84 visits)
(iii) The remainder are cytamen injections monthly (only 2 visits).

All of the above would be relatively short visits – allowing 10 minutes per visit – whereas a GNC may take 30–90 minutes. It can be seen, therefore, that although 5 and 7 need equal visits and have an equal number, this would bear no relation to the time needed to implement the care plan.

Rather than categorise patients by disease, the above groupings have been used; this is common practice by district nurses when allocating work. Terminal patients may therefore move from supervisory care (SV) when they are first referred to the service and subsequently to GNC as they become more dependent.

Performance appraisal

- Improve performance to improve effectiveness
- Increase the contribution of individual nurses
- Develop potential abilities to meet needs of service in future
- Top down approach
- Personality or performance?

It was felt that this was an extremely important principle to introduce into the service as it provided a positive strategy to help nurses achieve their goals and to facilitate professional development with individual nurses. However, before performance could be introduced effectively, there needed to be some work to provide an infrastructure for this to happen, firstly, the establishment of clinical supervision for the district nursing service. It was felt that this would provide a framework for performance appraisal especially in the light of the development of primary nursing. The work previously described on role definition of the district nurse as a nurse practitioner was dove-tailed at this stage into the framework.

Clinical supervision

Stewart and Sundeen (1993) suggest that experienced practitioners benefit just as much as more inexperienced ones from regular supervision; furthermore, Platt-Kosh (1986) suggests that within psychiatric nursing 'it is a disservice to both the patient and nurse to attempt to do psychiatric treatment without adequate clinical supervision' and concludes 'supervision is a valuable tool that the nurse therapist should use fully to develop the professional self.' With this in mind, a development model of clinical supervision was used, based on the following areas which were suggested by Stolenburg and Delworth (1987). It is tailored especially to the needs of the nurse seeking clinical supervision.

Educative   This component guides and facilitates knowledge transfer.

Supportive   This is a method by which clinical supervision enables the individual being supervised to perform clinical nursing skills in a controlled environment with support of the supervisor.

Managerial   This function enables the supervisor to assist the *supervisee* to acquire clinical managerial skills, gives feedback about the professional nursing skills and helps them to correct possible inadequacies. This theoretical construct parallels Benner's theory on the continuum of novice to expert.

Having established a model for clinical supervision, a performance appraisal system was implemented based on the following checklist:

- Improve performance to improve effectiveness.
- Increase the contribution of individual nurses.
- Develop potential abilities to meet needs of service in future.
- Top down approach.
- Personality or performance?

Conclusion

In summary, it was felt that the key model helped this district nursing service embed the principles of audit within its culture and organisation by providing a planned systematic approach and a bottom up approach to quality assurance. It provided a combination of data retrieval methods, integrated it into all its nursing functions and strongly aligned nursing standards with the audit cycle.

In using this model to develop a uni-professional audit tool it becomes apparent that this can only be achieved by good inter-organisational relationships and the working together of all professionals. Calman and Moores (NHS Management Executive, 1993) identify the urgency of moving from uni-professional audit to clinical audit:

'Whilst uni-professional audit will continue to have an important role, it has increasingly been realised that because the care of patients generally depends on the combined efforts of a number of professions the approaches to audit which are adopted need to reflect that fact.'

Therefore, the next step in working towards the goal of achieving this in the community, could be in the adaptation of the key model. The model would assist in the production of a collaborative or clinical audit tool which would bridge health and social care in the community.

The next stage in the audit process must, therefore, be a move to collaborative audit in the community, building on the long-standing good relationships with social service departments. Collaborative audit comes to the fore within the wider debate of joint purchasing and dissolving the boundaries between health markets and care markets. Work needs to be progressed on auditing across the health social care boundaries using perhaps nursing as the benchmark for good practice, based on nurses' track record in the use of audit.

References

Badger F, Cameron E and Evers H (1989) District nurses' patients – issues of caseload management. *Journal of Advanced Nursing* **14** (7): 518–527.
Benner P (1984) *From Novice to Expert*. California: Addison Wesley.
Calman K and Moores Y (1993) *Clinical Audit – Meeting and Improving Standards in Health Care*. London: HMSO.
Christoffel T and Lowenthall M (1977) Evaluating the quality of ambulatory health care – a review of emerging methods. *Medical Care* **XV** (11): 877–96.
Department of Health (1989) *Community Care: An Agenda for Action* (Griffiths Report). London: HMSO.
Evers H, Badger F, Cameron E and Atkin K (1988) *District Nursing, The Disabled and the Elderly: where are the black patients?* Community Care Project Working Papers, Health Services Research Unit, University of Birmingham.
Green C (1993) Teaching strategies for the process of planned change. *Journal of Continuing Education in Nursing* **14** (6): 16–23.
Groves T (1992). Countdown to community care – what the changes mean. *British Medical Journal* **305**: 1489–1490.
Jackson C (1993) Community care, your role or mine. *Health Visitor* **66** (4): 124.

Lewin K (1951) *Field Theory in Social Science*. New York: Harper and Row.

Littlewood J (1985) *The Use of the Nursing Process by District Nurses*. Sheffield: Centre for the Study of Primary Care Report.

Morison M J (1992) Prompting the motivation to change – the role of facilitative leadership in quality assurance. *Professional Nurse* **7** (11): 715–718.

NHS Management Executive (1991) *Framework of Audit for Nursing Services*. London: HMSO.

NHS Management Executive (1993) *Clinical Audit – Meeting and improving standards in health care*, p 2. London: HMSO.

Parker M, Quinn J, Viehl M, McKinley A, Polich C, Detzner C, Hartwell S and Korn K (1990) Case management in rural areas; definition, clients, financing, staffing, and service delivery issues. *NURSEcon* **8**: 104.

Plant R (1987) *Managing Change and Making It Stick*. London: Fontana.

Platt-Koch L M (1986) Clinical supervision for psychiatric nurses. *Journal of Psycho-social Nursing* **26** (1): 7–15.

Shaw C D (1986) *Introducing Quality Assurance*, Paper No. 64. London: King's Fund.

Smith S (1993) All change. *Nursing Times* **89** (3), January 20: 24–26.

Stewart G W and Sundeen S J (1993) *Principles and Practice of Psychiatric Nursing*, 2nd Edn. St. Louis: CV Mosby Co.

Stolenburg C D and Delworth U (1987) *Supervising Counsellors and Therapists*. San Francisco: Jossey-Bass.

UKCC (1992) *Scope of Professional Practice*. London: United Kingdom Central Council for Nursing, Midwifery and Health Visiting.

Yorkshire Health (1992) *Achieving Best Nursing Practice – Briefing for purchasers*. Yorkshire Regional Health Authority.

6

The Manager's Role in Audit

Management and the clinical professions

The NHS has traditionally consisted of clinical staff involved in patient care, and managers who have tended to 'manage the buildings' but who have not been very involved in clinical issues. The terms 'administrator', 'hospital secretary' and 'house governor' reflected this supporting role. Doctors, in their role as treaters of the sick and researchers, have tended to dominate decision making about patient care, and thus general service development. This has been largely due to their higher professional status relative to managers, nurses and other health care professionals. However, although doctors have led aspects of care such as diagnosis and treatment, there has been little coordinated management of individual patient's experience of their whole health care experience. This is partly due to the professionals' inability to assign a leading role in a consensus vacuum.

The 1974 reorganisation of the health service had introduced a unification of services, coordination between health authorities and local government and, lastly, 'consensus management'. The weaknesses of consensus at micro and macro levels in the NHS led to the introduction of general management as part of the Griffiths Report (1983). This reorganisation focused on decentralisation, and separated those services that 1974 had sought to unify. However, it was essentially consensus management, combined with the constant stream of central directives lacking direction, that was seen by Griffiths to be the root of the NHS institutional stalemate. The symptoms of this stalemate were delays in decision making, an elaborate consultation process and structural complexity. The report saw general management as providing leadership; achieving innovation and cost improvement; motivating staff; bringing professional judgement into the parameters of service objectives; and instigating efficient and effective consultation.

The importance of management was further accentuated in the 1989 reforms that gave greater freedom to provider units in the form of NHS Trusts, and thus to the general managers (chief executives) to manage the business of the Trusts, which is essentially the clinical services that the

Trust provides. The chief executive role gives the senior manager more responsibility for clinical matters and greater status within the organisation. The need to attract referrals in the form of contracts, and to perform against those contracts, prompts the manager to take a greater interest in clinical activity. The Trust board also holds the consultants' contracts, making the doctors locally accountable for their performance.

This change has coincided with some degree of challenge to the consultants' status. They have moved away from being clearly the first amongst equals, with associated clinical independence and freedom, to being more closely associated with service delivery in total, including the management of resources.

Traditionally, the consultant had defined and planned a clinical service and advised management on appropriate standards. Now, general practitioners and health authority purchasers are beginning to assert themselves, and express their views regarding the type, quantity and quality of services they require through the contracting process. The consultant now acts as a service provider, responding to clients' demands, and negotiating his/her position in relation to clinical expectations and desires. Clinical autonomy now exists within a tighter framework which seeks to advocate on the patient's behalf. This clearly compromises the previous position where clinical expertise was the prime factor in shaping care delivery. That expertise is now contextualised within resources and patients' expectations. The other health care professionals have also been affected by these roles. Nurses, who make up the largest staff group in the NHS, have traditionally suffered lower status, associated with the fact that they are predominantly women. Nursing is perceived as not having a discrete body of knowledge and that the work undertaken by nurses is profoundly personal and, in many instances, labelled as 'dirty' or naturally women's caring work.

General management heralded the end of the natural succession of nurses to middle and senior management positions. The traditional hierarchy of nursing was broken down as it became the norm for nurses to be managed by general managers from a variety of backgrounds, but commonly from a non-clinical base. It was not unusual for the ward sister to be managed by a non-nurse, and to have a second line of professional accountability to a director of nursing. This position was further challenged with the instigation of clinical directorates. While, in theory, the post of clinical director could be taken by any clinical professional, in reality, these posts were part of a wider agenda to involve doctors in management and thus in resource management. Nurses competed for business manager posts to support clinical directors, reinforcing the traditional picture of doctor (male) being supported in his decision making by nurses (female). Moreover, in many instances this structure weakened the nurse's contribution to board level decision making. At the same time, resource constraints meant that nursing staffing levels (the most expensive single outlay of any hospital) were also coming under review, with the inception of the nursing support worker. Nurses, therefore, are used to being managed by non-nurses, and to being scrutinised by other professionals. This has meant that nurses have had to learn to review their practice in a more visible and accountable way than medicine. The nursing contribution to service delivery has been recognised in the nurse executive role at Trust board level, mandatory within the reforms, which provides an opportunity for a stronger voice from nursing.

The status and standing of the paramedical professions has changed over the years. Following the 1974 reorganisation, many professions established a district head of service with direct access to the senior manager. However, the NHS reforms turned the table on this trend, with the professions allied to medicine (PAMs) having no mandatory representation at senior level. More commonly, the PAMs are subsumed within other services or clinical directorates and are managed by another professional. There has been a parallel development in the delivery of care. Instead of simply delivering available resources, professionals have been encouraged through the advent of resource management to assess patient needs before delivering treatment and care, and to evaluate outcomes.

Audit

Audit has emerged as a key aspect of performance evaluation. In Donabedian (1966) terms it has involved the review of inputs, process and outputs, with all acting, to some degree, as proxies for outcomes. The reason for this is primarily the difficulty in directly measuring outcomes of clinical treatment or care, or of service delivery. Ideally audit should capture the patient's whole experience of treatment, care and wider service delivery and should not be dominated by any one group of professionals, or concentrate on that professional group's inputs or process. Rather, audit should be multidisciplinary and should strive to become outcome focused. However, given the history of the NHS and the fight between the various interested parties to gain rank and status, it is hardly surprising that the recent audit initiative should have been medically led. Critics would say that it has also been kept secret to the medical profession, by hiding behind the ethical shield of accountability to protect medical interests.

Medical audit

The recent audit initiative sponsored by the NHS Management Executive (NHSME) has been medically led at every level of the service. The funding has been handed down from the NHSME to the regional medical directors, and then to local medical audit committees. The line of communication for audit has been between the regional health authority, and medical consultants with little involvement of local managers or other professions. The official guidance within Working Paper 6 (1989) states:

> The overall form of audit should be agreed locally between the profession and management, which itself needs to know that an effective system of medical audit is in place and that the work of each medical team is reviewed at regular and frequent intervals to be agreed locally.

and:

> The committee will produce an annual forward programme for medical audit within the district, to be agreed with the district general manager.

Moreover HC (91) 2 Medical Audit states:

> The committee will also provide regular reports to both medical staff and management . . . a broad outline of the aggregated results . . . together with any comparisons available . . . an account of any problems with data retrieval or analysis . . . an indication of action being taken or recommended. . . .

This has put management in a passive role as recipients of previously professionally screened findings with a uni-professional approach to solutions, which may well impact on the wider service. Experience of managers has varied greatly between providers, in terms of their active involvement in medical audit, and the impact of medical audit in service provision. However, many managers have felt excluded from the audit process, often on the basis or a suspected pretext that detailed results must be kept confidential.

Clearly, individual patient data should be subject to confidentiality, as should the honest self-criticism of doctors whose professional practice is subject to audit. Otherwise, the danger is that audit becomes a threat and those being audited become defensive, looking for justification of their actions rather than for improvements. Clearly, a balance has to be struck between respecting the confidentiality of the patient and subjecting audit results to a wider scrutiny in order to make the best improvements in the patient's whole experience. Thus, much of audit could be shared within healthcare. The general public may well be reassured to know that such rigorous self and peer analysis is taking place.

Professional resistance to a more open approach might be seen as simply doctors acting as a trade union and exerting their undoubted political strength within the NHS. They could be accused of doing this to defend their present position and to ensure that audit does not threaten the interests of the profession or individual doctors. Obviously, detailed examination of personal professional practice is a sensitive issue. However, many places have taken the line that audit is a delicate flower, to the extent that there is a danger that proper supervision of the audit process has not taken place and it has become a professional preserve for doctors only.

Involving managers in the audit process

A District Medical Audit Committee should be established. . . . together with doctor(s) representing the District General Manager. (Working Paper 6, 1989)

In some places the director of public health (pre-reforms) has been involved, as a proxy for managerial involvement, but has not necessarily fully briefed the general manager. This situation should not be seen in isolation. Only recently (1990) have general managers had a say in the appointment of consultants working in their unit. However, the system of merit awards for consultants (which can double their salary and thus have a significant impact on the Trust's budget) is secretive in the extreme. General managers have little say in the awards as they are based on publications and research, i.e. contribution to the advancement of the field of medical knowledge, not on performance in terms of the putting theory into practice, or contribution to service delivery.

By contrast, the Royal Colleges have a formal, strong influence on many local medical matters. For example, the right to approve junior posts for training gives them an opportunity to impose standards for consultant numbers, bed numbers, and the detail of on-call rotas at all levels. As a result, although the picture is changing, managers have in many ways been marginalised in terms of their ability to manage consultants and medical matters for many years. As such, there is a precedent for their minimal involvement in audit. However, it is also fair comment to say that many managers do not take a real interest in medical and clinical matters (how many regularly read a clinical journal?) and have failed to show a proper interest in any clinical or medical audit.

A key recent development is that the reforms have brought a split between purchaser and provider, with many public health doctors remaining on the health authority/purchaser side. This has meant that within Trusts there is now the potential for the medical director (who is more inclined than a public health doctor to take a hands-on approach to operational issues) to become more involved in the management of the Trust and in the delivery of audit. In some Trusts, the medical director chairs the audit committee. This can provide an effective lead to audit, as long as consultants can accept the strong managerial link and are reassured with regard to appropriate confidentiality arrangements.

The future for medical audit

Some evidence is now emerging that the confidential, voluntary system has not worked well. It has certainly been patchy, with mixed results between and within units. Some specialities in some hospitals appear to be relatively inactive. Attendance rates vary and many do not use the full session available. There must be a real question mark against the value for money of medical audit, since the investment in both money and medical time is substantial and there is little evidence as yet of 'the audit loop being closed' to the significant benefit of patients or the organisation. It appears, therefore, that a firmer approach is required with clear objectives being set. Equally, it has to be recognised that if audit is too external, and threatening, then doctors will simply become defensive and use audit to re-affirm existing practice, rather than using it to its full potential to improve clinical practice.

Clearly, there is a need to take a more positive approach. The changing nature in the relationship between managers and doctors puts managers in a slightly stronger position. For example, Trust status involves Trusts in holding consultants' contracts, and the chief executive and medical director, while limited in their real authority, are at least more closely and locally involved in consultants' activities. In another sense, managers certainly need to be involved to help close the 'feedback loop'. Some audit findings will require managerial activity to resolve non-clinical problems (e.g. poor engineering standards) or management directed resources (e.g. funding a new kitchen or an additional nurse post).

Nationally there has also been the move towards reviews of particular services and clinical practice including:

CEPOD (confidential enquiry into perioperative deaths)
CESDI (confidential enquiry into still births and deaths in infancy)
MTOS (major trauma outcome study)

Unfortunately the response rate to CEPOD is less than 20 per cent, but it does show that those patients receiving specialist attention fare better and that there is room for improvement in many areas (Maynard, 1993). These reports have raised issues as to the appropriate mix of work within specialities at district general hospital level, and have prompted the need for audit to justify existing practice. However, as yet, purchasers have not taken up the challenge to build in requirements to be informed of the results of these studies, which would put pressure on providers to ensure doctors take part in the studies and provide an incentive to improve their results. This may be addressed as funding for audit moves to purchasers. In future, audit will be funded through contracts from purchasers to providers, which will lead to purchasers beginning to take an interest in audit, specifying topics, and expecting some feedback.

Doctors and managers: common goals?

Doctors and managers are actually motivated to want to achieve the same result of better patient care, both in terms of individual care and total care delivered. Doctors have a more direct commitment to individual care, since their predominant role lies in individual patient contact and care. Inevitably, they will want to optimise clinical quality, with possibly less regard to overall resource use. Managers may tend to generalise, to take a broader view, and thereby seem to disregard individual patient care. Audit for doctors may, therefore, represent the maintenance of professional standards and standing, whereas managers may want to use it to streamline services and to challenge doctors' performance. Inevitably, there are potential tensions in such differing values.

Developing clinical audit

Audit should of course be applied to all areas of work. Logically, it should be driven by services delivered to users not by professional group. So far, managers have failed to support both medical audit and audit initiatives in other areas. Nurses have pressed for both nursing and clinical audit but with little response in many cases. Managers have not been encouraged to support them or to invest the necessary finance. The Department of Health has invested some money in nursing and therapy audit but it is a small amount compared with the investment in medical audit. Clearly this has caused some frustration and has been a lost opportunity. The other professions are also beginning to recognise the need for audit and to exercise their independence. Again, managers have not shown the necessary response. However, the time is now ripe to develop clinical audit, as all levels of staff within provider units recognise the need to audit their performance in order to assure purchasers of the quality of their healthcare. This coincides with greater attempts to measure outcomes and other indicators of performance.

The Department of Health is now actively encouraging and supporting clinical audit, and there has been a clear shift of emphasis in that direction with the launch of the policy statement *Clinical Audit* (Department of Health, 1993). This policy heralds the last year of separate funding, combining medical, nursing and therapy audit allocations into one allocation for clinical audit from 1994.

Managerial interests

In principle, managers' actions should be driven by the business plan for the organisation. The provider corporate agenda now clearly includes

delivering on contracts with purchasers. Traditionally, the NHS has func-
tioned around referrals from GPs to consultants. However, consultants
were in effect funded direct to deliver services and determined, through
their own professional advice, the most appropriate service. The Reforms
have had a dramatic impact. Purchasers, with GP advice, now contract with
providers to deliver services. This relationship involves discussion about
both cost and quality, with the latter beginning to incorporate clinical
issues. Provider managers are then obliged to deliver on such contracts,
and consultants have moved more towards being deliverers of services
rather than the determiners of those services. Provider managers are
prompted to be concerned about delivering their contracts and, therefore,
about the clinical elements within those contracts. Progressively, purchasers and providers will begin to focus on these clinical components,
which will include clinical outcomes.

Part of this will derive from the national issues revolving around, for
example, the appropriate location for more specialist surgery and a general
need to demonstrate excellent or acceptable performance. Similarly, purchasers will seek assurance that 'state of the art' services are being
provided. Provider managers will want to demonstrate excellence to
enhance their competitive edge in the market. The managers themselves
now see the need for much more audit activity and have begun to recognise
the need for such investment, although there is still some reticence due to
the competing pressures on limited budgets.

The issue of audit confidentiality

Medical audit has been carried out within a strong atmosphere of secrecy.
There have even been debates on whether managers should be notified if
poor practice by a doctor is discovered and not corrected. The technical
position on the sharing of information is as follows:

> The results of medical audit in respect of individual patients and doctors
> must remain confidential at all times. However, the general results need to be
> made available to local management so that they may be able to satisfy
> themselves that appropriate remedial action is taken where audit results
> reveal problems. (Working Paper 6, Para 3.2.d, 1989)

In practice, the degree of anonymity and abstraction has made it difficult
for managers to take action and has, in fact, demotivated managers from
exploiting the full potential benefits of medical audit. As clinical audit
begins to take over from medical audit, results will be more public. The
other professions have less inclination to secrecy and managers will be in a
stronger position to determine the policy. Undoubtedly, more information
will be made available to purchasers and they are likely to demand this

through contracts for audit as purchasers take over the responsibility for audit funding from regional health authorities. In practice, this information may be fed to the director of public health rather than the chief executive. This alone moves audit results closer to the public domain. However, specific medical audit by a named doctor will and should continue to be supported by the appropriate degree of confidentiality and anonymity.

A theoretical but hopefully rare issue in practice is: what if dangerous practice by an individual doctor is identified through audit? In practice, either formally or informally, one trusts the audit chairman would notify management; it is, however, an issue that has caused some anxiety.

Focus of audit

In some units, the core issues of medical practice have given way to the more comfortable review of peripheral issues such as the quality of medical records, and issues around junior doctor performance.

Sometimes this has been accompanied by a downgrading of the status of membership of the audit committee, such that attendance is more a burden for the most junior consultant within a speciality rather than a responsibility carried by more senior consultants. There now needs to be a revitalisation of the system. Whether clinical or medical, there must be a clear focus on the challenging issues, where change is required, and implementation may not be easy. While some 'housekeeping' style checks are appropriate to be sure that general systems are working properly, it is the concerns, deficiencies, and questionable practice that should be challenged through audit. Minor examples include whether general anaesthetics or sedation should be used for colonoscopies and whether surgical shaves and 'skin preps' are required pre-operatively. Local practice varies between consultants without apparent due cause. In some cases, such as surgical shaves, there is clear research-based evidence as to better practice, which needs implementation. In some instances this is an audit function, in others it is more to do with the need simply to update and improve practice. Audit can, however, help highlight problems.

More significantly, do surgical complication rates vary between doctors? Do survival rates vary for life threatening diseases? Is best practice being used in terms of chemotherapy and pharmaceutical regimes? (e.g. for breast cancer and cardiac arrest, respectively). In the former case, audit overlaps with research and development, in the latter, with the issue of measuring outcomes.

Managerial role in effecting change through the audit cycle

The relevant quote from Working Paper 6, Para 3.3, (1989) is as follows:

> While the practice of medical audit is essentially a professional matter management too has significant responsibility for seeing that resources are used in the most effective way, and will therefore need to ensure that an effective system of medical audit is in place.

Management needs to ensure that effective audit is taking place and support doctors, nurses and therapists in terms of implementing change. Management should help resolve difficulties in cross-departmental audit, e.g. pressure sores identified on wards, due to slow accident and emergency department throughput and admission to wards, or due to old mattresses well past their sell-by date. Management should also identify issues for audit projects, e.g. do budgets devolved to wards help improve clinical care?

An interesting issue is the monitoring of clinical outcomes. Managers may well feel this is a legitimate corporate concern which may be best handled through the audit system.

Using audit to improve clinical quality

Due to the very limited feedback, in general, about audit, there is little evidence of its impact on quality. In principle, audit can also be used to try to resolve specific perceived problems. Technically, the audit framework facilitates this:

> Where necessary management must be able to initiate an independent audit. This may take the form of external peer review or a joint professional and managerial appraisal of a particular service. (Working Paper 6, Para 3.2.e, 1989)

Such audit can be used to look at issues of poor techniques and poor facilities. It can look at the need for new technology and whether new technology is being effectively used.

Specifically, audit can be used to address the problem of clinicians who may be working below an acceptable clinical level of performance. The local manager can initiate a review:

> Where there is unresolved concern about a particular service, the committee may initiate an independent review, or the general manager may ask it to do so. (Working Paper, Para 11, 6)

Audit and information technology

Good audit needs good information and the ideal is to use routinely collected data (i.e. used for other purposes) which is 'owned' by clinical staff. Traditionally, available data have been poor (clerks recording gynaecology procedures for male patients etc). Collecting basic data solely for audit is time consuming.

Part of the audit funding, in terms of capital, has been for the acquisition of computer systems. Proliferation of incompatible systems within specialties must be avoided; the ideal is to use systems linked to 'patient administration' type systems. Resource management systems offer the potential to provide case-mix data, plus more specific data for individual specialties, but it is still early days in terms of assessing the effectiveness of this approach.

Audit and quality

Proponents of quality in the NHS have tended to shy away from clinical areas. Audit should now be used as a complementary tool, to provide quality assurance and quality improvement in the clinical heartland. A related issue is that of patient satisfaction. Managers have felt able to ask patients about the car parking and the food and even about nursing care. However, patients' views on their clinical care and the way it is delivered are often not ascertained, due to resistance from doctors. Clearly it is relevant and could provide useful audit data.

Research and teaching

Audit should be 'research-based' but should not involve major research activity – it is about assuring good practice, not developing it. However, the introduction of new and better practice and equipment must be part of the managerial agenda and can provide a bridge between research and audit. It is obvious that implementing research should improve clinical performance and this is also a desired aim of audit. The best overlap is when research prompts new practice and audit is used to ensure that the new practice works and secures the desired benefits.

Risk management

Risk management is about the identification of significant risks within an organisation, and the action taken to address those risks. Clearly, risky clinical practice is common ground between audit and risk management. A key managerial role should be to use audit results to inform risk analysis and use risk reports (patterns of incidents etc) to prompt audit work. Many Trusts now find it helpful to have a risk management committee. This approach does imply a sharing of information for the common good and effective data collection and reporting on both sides. In practical terms cross-membership of committees is helpful.

Audit and accreditation

A development in parallel to audit is that of accreditation. While in the UK we do not yet have formal accreditation, the King's Fund organisational audit initiative moves us in that direction. The King's Fund project involves voluntary participation in a whole organisation review, including a visit by a team of trained inspectors. Much of the preparation work involves making sure that there are well-documented policies and procedures in a whole range of areas covered by checklists.

Organisational audit and other such initiatives move the NHS towards formal accreditation of providers and, possibly, consultants. The former, or both, could face formal review and assessment on a periodic basis, to be licensed to deliver healthcare. Documented use of clinical audit would then almost certainly be required.

Protocols

Much work is being invested in developing care protocols or similar approaches which involve the specification and documentation of packages of healthcare. These are intended to help clinical staff in their approach to individual patients. 'Case management' can be used to ensure that patient treatment adheres to the protocol. They can include supportive policies, advising on good or best practice (how to catheterise etc) and protocols intended to control use of resources (laboratory testing guidelines etc).

All such protocols can be used to form a valuable baseline for audit, since much local practice is actually based on a verbal tradition and, as such, is difficult to identify, measure, audit and improve. Many of the shortcomings identified once protocols are implemented and monitored relate to 'system' as opposed to 'people' failings. Managers can have a key role to play in making sure that the right processes are in place and that these are properly supported with appropriate back-up. Once more, audit, through protocols, can identify organisational shortcomings. It is then often a management role to 'close the feedback loop' and make necessary changes. (For more information on protocols see Chapter 3.)

Resources to support audit

Specific funding has been allocated by the Department of Health over recent years and has included capital allocations as well as revenue.

However, medical audit has been slow to get off the ground. The ring fencing of the funding could have ensured prompt action, but handling funding and development outside the general management line has led to a lack of drive and certainty with regards to development. The capital that has been made available has been spent very slowly and there is a suspicion that it has been used on IT equipment which may well be intended, at least partly, for other use. There is, however, still a linked problem regarding capital investment to provide offices for audit staff. Most providers will have an audit person for each speciality who needs office space. This is not a straightforward issue, given the lack of office space for consultants and junior doctors. The revenue is intended mainly for staff but, due to lack of local management involvement, there has been real uncertainty as to whether the funding is long term. As a result, there has been a tendency only for short-term appointments to be made, to the detriment of the initiative.

There is a real need to ensure that proper long-term appointments are made and that capital is properly invested (no new capital is being allocated, but there is a backlog). The appropriate guidance already exists:

> Health Authorities and managers have a responsibility to ensure that appropriate resources are available to support audit programmes. (Health Circular (91) 2)

It should be remembered, and managers are only too well aware, that there are two substantial costs to audit. One is the direct funding, the other is the time invested by clinicians in carrying out audit. Most providers have a system of rotating half days dedicated to medical audit activity. The norm is one half day per month, which equates to 2.5 per cent of medical time. Clearly this is a substantial resource and must be used effectively. Separate time has not been made available to the other professions. Nurses and therapists are expected to fit audit in to their everyday work, without a decrease in clinical activity. Audit then becomes subject to short-term priorities, such as clinical crisis, sickness, bereavement and so on.

Funding for clinical audit

Some funds are now being made available to support small initiatives involving joint audit between doctors and other clinicians. For example, bids have recently been requested for community orientated clinical audit. However, a significant development in audit for other professions will require significant investment. Medical audit alone costs around 0.5 per cent of revenue to fund the staffing. Clearly, clinical audit will cost at least as much again for proper support. The real problem though may well be making staff time available on a regular basis, if dedicated time is used.

Better and more focused use of ward rounds and nurse handovers could provide some audit time, but more will be needed to provide resources to help change practice once problems are identified. Alternatively, it may be possible to carry out good audit using time opportunistically.

Incentives to participate in audit

Some doctors have participated fully and enthusiastically, but many have not. It may be sufficient to make audit mandatory as real self-analysis in professional terms needs voluntary participation. However, logically, audit participation should be a key objective for individuals and could be linked to remuneration. Presently, for doctors, the option is to try to tie eligibility for merit awards to audit. For other staff, individual performance review (IPR) and performance-related pay could be used to foster audit activities. Recognition for clinical supervision could be an option, linked to some remuneration.

There is an issue as to whether clinical audit results should be included in IPR reviews. For a ward sister, a high pressure sore rate (e.g. due to poor patient assessment, handwashing etc) would warrant a lower rating. Certainly this would put nursing care back into performance review mechanisms that have become dominated by management ability and skills. Although audit may not be intended directly to save money, it could be that any savings achieved through audit could be fed back to individual budgets to provide some incentive.

Purchaser and provider roles

The NHS reforms have separated managerial roles into purchasing ('commissioning') and provision. So far, this chapter has concentrated on the provider managerial role, where the manager has a direct interest in ensuring that excellent clinical services are delivered locally.

Purchasers have a distinct role in terms of concentrating on the health needs of the population. They place contracts with providers to deliver appropriate healthcare. They then have a legitimate interest in 'quality assuring' those contracts. One element to that is the clinical content and quality. Therefore, purchasers are beginning to seek information about audit and, through their own doctors (directors of public health), some access to the clinical results. This will overlap with their developing interest in monitoring outcomes and should provide a healthy stimulus to audit activity. Moreover, despite differences of interest, audit is one area where provider managers are keen to have purchaser interest to support their own wish to increase audit activity.

Audit in non-clinical areas

Audit is also relevant in other areas, as part of a systematic review of performance. Organisation audit, BS5750 applications, and other accreditation activities prompt assessment and audit of processes and performance. Thus, for example, the Yorkshire Health Estates department uses a quality manual and audit tool to monitor standards and performance.

Audit of audit

Little work has been done so far in terms of whether audit is value for money. Managers would wish to monitor audit but need access to more detail with regards to individual studies to assess effectiveness. It would appear to be ripe for an Audit Commission review.

Conclusion

Harman and Martin (1992) identify two roles for managers in audit:

1. Supporting medical audit, through the provision of information and resources.
2. Managing the integration of medical audit into the corporate workings of the Trust by creating a climate for audit and establishing the parameters in which audit takes place.

Another role identified in this chapter is the instigator of audit, for areas of concern to clients, non-executives, the Trust board or the chief executive. The chief executive's prime objective is to secure the viability and success of the Trust through successful marketing of its capabilities. This requires collaboration between all professional groups to ensure the best use of resources to achieve the best outcomes for patients. It also requires a shared understanding of professional aspirations, and potential within the market. While tension between professional groups can produce critical review, it is vital that managers seek to build and support multidisciplinary teams that are able actively to plan service developments based on research and systematic audit. This requires professionals to work in partnership with managers towards common goals.

References

Department of Health and Social Security (1983) *Report of the Management Inquiry* (Griffiths Report). London: HMSO.

Department of Health (1989) *Working for Patients: Working paper 6*. London: HMSO.

Department of Health (1991) *HC (91) 2: Medical Audit in the Hospital and Community Health Services*. London: HMSO.

Department of Health (1993) *Clinical Audit*. Lancs: The Health Publications Unit.

Donabedian A (1966) Evaluating the quality of medical care. *Milbank Memorial Fund Quarterly* **44** (3), part 2: 166–206.

Harman D and Martin G (1992) Managers and medical audit. *The Health Services Journal*, April, 27–29.

Maynard A (1993) A great leap forward. *The Health Services Journal*, 15 July, 23.

7

Breaking Down Professional Boundaries

Introduction

Patient care is focused through multidisciplinary and multiprofessional teamwork in most clinical specialties in an attempt to minimise its fragmentation. It is impossible to isolate the contribution of one professional group when looking at patient outcomes, as the reality is that high quality care is seldom achieved by people from a single discipline. The outcomes of care will depend on the contribution and cooperation of a group of health care staff.

However, in a contrast to this, health care professionals often act as a 'community within a community' (Surgeon, 1990) with distinctive and integrated occupational cultures. They have a common sense of identity, a shared conscience on their social role and a common language. McKenna (1992) points out that strict lines of professional demarcation make no sense since patients cross them all the time. Patients themselves do not understand the different professional tribal associations; poor quality of care given by any one professional could sour the entire experience for the patient.

Questions should therefore be asked about the extent to which professionals put their own occupational interests before those of the patients. It is generally accepted that doctors, nurses and therapists should work in cooperation to maximise the quality of care given to patients. Mackay (1993) suggests that such collaboration could be achieved by getting professionals to understand and appreciate the stresses and strains of their colleagues.

The apparent failure to appreciate the stresses of colleagues' work may stem partly from generalised perceptions of the other occupations (Mackay, 1993). For example, nurses are seen as handmaidens of the medical profession, from which it may follow that all that nurses do is to tidy, clean and wipe bottoms. Likewise, it may be perceived that all that physiotherapists do is get patients out of bed and show them how to walk. Such stereotypes can critically affect working relationships.

Schools of nursing and medicine have played a major part in the acquisition of culture and values that fit in with these stereotypes (Simpson, 1979) of the dominant–subservient relationship between doctors and nurses (Stein, 1967). McKenna (1992) comments that this professional isolation begins during training, as there is no common curriculum for the various groups of students of health care. Wright (1985) comments that no single health service profession can provide all the knowledge or resources required for total patient care, and yet there has been little progress towards setting up multidisciplinary training in this country. Participation in a joint introduction to clinical studies may begin to help students understand the roles and contributions of other professions and so help to demonstrate the philosophy that no single discipline has all the solutions. Many professionals would very much like to have their stresses and workload appreciated by their colleagues.

Currently, the picture of the ideal colleague is built up from a number of different sources, including socialisation before entering an occupation and socialisation within it. Images of role models are then built upon positive reinforcement by the power brokers of particular sets of behaviours exhibited during working life. For many such power brokers (e.g. consultants) their power depends on the traditional *status quo* being reinforced; thus, any attempts to find alternative behaviours more appropriate to modern society and to health care requirements, fall on stony ground. An example of this can be seen in the Department of Health initiative to reduce junior doctors' hours. While junior doctors are supportive, there are instances where consultants believe that the reduction in hours will compromise the juniors' clinical experience, or that the enhancement of nursing roles should be constrained to the mundane and repetitive duties that juniors currently carry out, rather than to a shift in responsibility for care management.

The division between health care professionals is perhaps most clearly reinforced by the separate patient records each of them complete for patients within their care. A single patient record would begin to show the degree of collaboration between the professions and make multidisciplinary quality assurance easier. In order to do this there would need to be a common understanding of patients' rights in terms of access, ownership and contribution to their records. An example of where this does appear to have been solved is in pregnancy, where the mother carries her own records at all times, and in the advent of parent-held records in paediatrics.

Currently, within the NHS, there is another group which is having an effect on the work of doctors, nurses and therapists – that of management, whose influence has substantially increased over the last few years. The establishment of clinical directorates has devolved responsibility for budgets down to units, with a large amount of power being held by the budget holder. To some extent, this has had less effect on nurses and therapists than on doctors, who have not in the past been subject to managerial review, let alone to structured performance management. The ability of all health care professions to resist changes in operational activities has been reduced. For example, nurses have, in many areas, lost managerial control over nurses and there may be no-one to support them or their interests at the most senior management level. Equally, the increasing emphasis on value for money and quality of service means that the autonomy of the medical profession will be lessened as the practices of doctors come under closer scrutiny (Mackay, 1993). Working together to measure the quality of their patient care may be a step towards re-balancing the power game between professionals and management. Moreover, it is vital in terms of surviving the market for managers and clinical professionals to work together towards the Trust's corporate objectives. This serves the interests of the managers, clinical professionals and patients as it secures contracts to support the work of the Trust and should improve the quality of care the patient receives. Managers often feel that the clinical professionals work at odds to these corporate objectives, in striving for personal clinical excellence or for advancements in the clinical field. Surviving in the market requires all sides to work together to meet contractual obligations, while developing services within the market.

However, not only is there an imbalance of power between professionals and management, there is also an unequal distribution of power between the health care professions themselves. In most instances, it is doctors who decide which patients are admitted to hospital and when, how long they will stay and what the main focus of their treatment will be. This gives doctors a great deal of control over the work of nurses and therapists. The rise of the nurse practitioner, and the development of nursing or therapy beds, is beginning to demonstrate that the patient's primary need may not be for medical intervention. Many health services operate respite care beds and rehabilitative beds for the chronic sick and elderly. These remain in the minority and do not attract the glamour or the resources of consultant-managed beds.

Historically, the medical profession has maintained control over the role of the nurse by the adoption of the medical model in nurse education. This model developed from the Crimean War, when the army doctors taught Florence Nightingale's nurses how to carry out tasks and the skills they needed to support their work. This enabled the nurses to take on duties which had previously been carried out by the doctors. These were undertaken alongside the caring functions so valued by Miss Nightingale. Following the Second World War, the nurse's role moved towards those areas of clinical practice which brought the nurse into close contact with doctors and medical technology. Nurses then began to take on more tasks which the doctor no longer wished to carry out. His permission to take on the tasks was required as was his knowledge base and so medicine again increased its control over the development of the role of the nurse (White, 1988). In fact, doctors had a great deal of power and control over what nurses learned and, indeed, which of them subsequently qualified, as the doctors often organised the nursing examinations. A 'good' nurse was seen as one who carried out the doctor's orders accurately and efficiently, perhaps regardless of the patient care outcome (Keddy *et al.*, 1986). It is common today for doctors to lecture to nurses during their pre- and postregistration courses. It is much rarer for nurses to be seen lecturing doctors on knowledge specific to nursing.

The professions allied to medicine have managed to achieve some autonomy and independence from the medical profession. The inclusion of non-medical subjects in the curriculum and the development of degree courses have meant that medical control over the knowledge of therapists has been challenged. This challenge will only become a reality when therapy services are not dependent on the referral of a doctor but can accept referrals from any health care professional, or self-referral from the patient.

Nursing began to move towards similar autonomy with the arrival of the nursing process in the 1970s. However, this was interpreted in some medical areas as an open threat to their traditional dominance (Wright, 1985). Some doctors saw the 'process' as being deliberately used to exclude them from nursing affairs, resulting in a threat to the *status quo* of the doctor–nurse relationship as nurses began to increase their own knowledge and skills, more clearly defining their own role with regard to patient care but without necessarily following 'doctor's orders'. Nurses had begun to define the unique elements of their practice in contributing to the patient's progress.

Nurses and therapists carry out work which is less prestigious in society's eyes than that of doctors. Primarily it is women's work and, to a certain extent, relies on expertise developed from experience and intuition. Moreover, it is work always attributed to the natural instincts of women, therefore requiring little preparation or expertise. Their roles have none of the apparent mystery of medicine and of the 'cure' which doctors can effect (Mackay, 1993) as it is holistic rather than scientific. The importance of comfort in contributing to a patient's recovery may be as vital or more vital than the investigative endoscopy and subsequent prescription carried out by the doctor. However, the public will always attribute greater importance to the physiological latter solution than to the less tangible former. Despite the code of professional practice requiring nurses to operate independently in their actions and to hold full accountability for those actions, much of nurse's time in the acute sector is dictated by the doctor handing down instructions. While the acute hospital service is the minority of the health service, as a whole it certainly attracts the most interest and a disproportionate amount of funding. This further mitigates against other health care professionals who dominate service provision in the community, at least in numbers if not in status.

However, the contribution to decision making about patient care does not rest solely with the doctors, despite appearances to the contrary. Stein (1967) described what he called 'the doctor–nurse game' in which nurses communicate what to do to doctors without appearing to do so. The nurse guides the doctor by hints and comments so that the doctor continues to appear to be in charge. This manipulation is seen by nurses to be in the patient's best interests as it results in patients getting the correct decision, without overtly challenging the doctor's authority. As a result, nurses accept that their knowledge and experience must not be displayed, so as not to reduce a patient's faith in the care and treatment they are receiving, or the doctor's personal pride as the 'expert'.

This relationship is as much about women's relationship with men as it is doctors' relationship with nurses and originates in the gender imbalance of the two professions. It was not until the 19th Century that medicine admitted women and membership of the Royal College of Nursing was only expanded to men in 1968. This imbalance has been dramatically reversed over the last 10 years, with medical school intake running at 50 per cent men and 50 per cent women. However, women in medicine (despite comparable performance) are still less successful than their male counterparts, partly due to the break afforded by child rearing and partly due to the difficulty women have in being appointed to high status consultant specialities (e.g. cardiac surgery). This change in gender balance, alongside the improvement of nurse and therapy education, has led to the situation where the Cinderella professions are no longer prepared to act out the handmaiden role in order to get their opinions considered. Nurses and therapists are setting themselves up as independent practitioners and as specialists in their own right.

The advent of primary nursing has challenged the routine of doctors and the inherent power they hold. This transference of power and increase in confidence amongst the traditionally female professions heralds a new relationship between the professionals. However, these relationships are still in their infancy, and in many places the traditional model resists change. New role development requires partnership and recognition of mutual worth. Audit, even more so, requires confidence and trust between the professionals.

Many of the recent quality initiatives within the health service have developed in professional isolation. Nurses became involved in quality assurance in the mid 1980s to maintain high quality care for their patients. A series of high-profile books and articles were published, together with courses and workshops, which resulted in a horde of clinical standards. The professions allied to medicine subsequently also went through a similar process. Medical audit finally entered the area in 1991.

McKenna (1992) suggests that medical audit is a form of 'quality assurance quarantine', where quarantine is 'isolation for medical reasons'. Some doctors are reluctant to involve other disciplines on the basis of professional independence and confidentiality. The Audit Commission (1991) found that medical audit was often held behind closed doors. Equally, nurses and therapists have expressed concern about medical staff automatically taking the lead in multidisciplinary audit, and that their own views and contributions may therefore be engulfed. Moreover, nurses in particular have a longer experience in the field of standard setting and do not take kindly to the discovery of standards by medicine, and the automatic professional superiority that can go with it. However, when faced with medical scrutiny, nurses and therapists quickly lose confidence in their own expertise. As nurses and therapists become more confident in auditing within their own professional groups, they will undoubtedly be willing to take on the challenge of multidisciplinary audit.

Initiatives in collaboration

There are now a number of initiatives developing within the Health Service in which groups of professionals work together to look at the overall care received by their patients. This section will discuss just a few of which the author has personal knowledge and experience.

The PA-RNOH Nursing Quality Measurement Scale

The Nursing Quality Measurement Scale is designed to assess the current quality of nursing care in wards and to provide the means for concentrating attention on those issues which will lead to improvements in quality. It was developed in the UK by a team of nursing and healthcare consultants and produces both a descriptive assessment and a numerical rating of quality. The tool is divided into five sections which include structure, process, outcome measures and action plans and forms the basis of a peer review audit, which is carried out by two clinically based nurses.

A number of interesting issues emerged from the introduction of the Nursing Quality Measurement Scale at the Royal National Orthopaedic Hospital, Stanmore. For example, looking at the practice of others has encouraged the assessors to become critical of their own practice and, in some areas, they have introduced change as a result of an audit they have carried out elsewhere in the hospital. It quickly became apparent that issues were being identified which were common to a number of wards, making it possible to give feedback to other departments (such as hotel services) that was relevant to all wards' experiences of these services. This meant that they were not contacted individually by each ward about the same problem.

The audit process also highlighted the fact that nursing cannot be isolated from other disciplines when measuring patient care quality. One aspect of this was that the assessors found difficulty in discounting the contribution made by paramedical and medical staff to patient care when they were sitting carrying out direct observations of care.

Relevant information gathered during the audits was reported back to both the physiotherapy and occupational therapy departments. This raised interest in the issue of audit within those departments and resulted in the Nursing Quality Measurement Scale being adapted for use in paramedical practice (Paramedical Quality Measurement Scale, unpublished). Much of the tool was able to be transferred with little alteration, particularly the sections concerned with assessing the department's resources and reviewing the patient documents.

However, the area which caused some difficulty in transition was that of the direct observation of paramedical work. A sizeable amount of work undertaken by paramedical staff occurs on the wards. While observing nursing care does not present too much of a problem, as the assessors sit and watch the care given to a group of patients over a period of time, the paramedical staff treat patients on a number of wards and there was a danger that the observers may have to follow a member of staff around the hospital. This raises the issues of both anonymity of staff during the audits and the unobtrusiveness, or otherwise, of the assessors. The assessors therefore carry out their observation in either the physiotherapy depart-ment or the wards, depending on the physiotherapist's workload and where her/his patients are mainly located. They do not focus on the physio-therapist's actual techniques of treatment but look instead at their patient skills, such as lifting and handling, communication, respect for the patient's dignity and privacy. Although the physiotherapists have found this quite threatening, they feel that the feedback they receive is of real value to them.

The next logical stage in the progression of the quality measurement scale is to develop an observation of multidisciplinary or total patient care. One of the main factors within this will be a decision as to who should observe and make judgements about the quality of care the patient receives. This is when professional 'tribalism' again rears its ugly head. Currently, nurses observe nursing care, physiotherapists observe physiotherapy treat-ments and occupational therapists observe occupational therapy. Incident-ally, no-one observes medical treatment. It is not feasible to have four or more people (one for each profession) sitting in a group watching the care received by a number of patients, as their presence within the ward would be conspicuous to say the least. The issue of healthcare professionals' inability to accept comments about their practice and patient care from members of other disciplines will therefore have to be resolved. In some respects, it could be argued that this would be a positive move, as the staff have not been socialised into other professions' accepted practices and so may be in a position to challenge or ask naive questions. The ultimate point of this discussion may be to examine the role patients may have to play in the observation of care. Could they perhaps be the best arbiters of what constitutes the best quality care?

Multidisciplinary plans of care

This approach is gaining interest in the UK under a number of different guises, such as critical paths, core care plans, care maps, anticipated recovery paths. They are all basically multidisciplinary tools which identify the care which should be given to a specific group of patients at agreed times during their stay in hospital and document this in one common record. In some instances, defined aspects of assessment of the patient can be done by any one of the professionals involved in the patient's care (e.g. social history, nutritional status, functional mobility). This ensures that the patient is not repeatedly asked the same question, that records are not duplicated and that the care team are working towards agreed goals/outcomes.

One of the main goals of multidisciplinary plans of care is to promote collaborative practice between nursing, paramedical and medical staff, through improved communication and understanding of the role of each of the team members in patient care. The plan should be drawn up and agreed by the multidisciplinary group responsible for the patient, with each group of staff involved in the patient's care represented. The group should appoint a coordinator of care (usually the nurse, as he/she is likely to spend the most time in direct contact with the patient and is the most accessible to the patient) to ensure that the care follows the agreed plan as closely as possible. However, each professional has a responsibility to ensure their own part is filled to the best of their ability.

Many hospitals which have taken one of these approaches have begun by looking at orthopaedics, as the care for many of these patients is relatively easy to define and plan. Other selective surgical procedures also lend themselves well to this approach. Complex pathology makes standardised pre-set plans of care difficult but should not prevent the principles of mutual assessment and goal setting. When used in practice, every member of staff who cares for the patient should contribute to the plan. Inevitably, however, much of the documentation falls to the nursing staff, an issue which may need further discussion within the multidisciplinary team. In achieving a common multidisciplinary record, the principles of ease of use, exception reporting and patient recording will lead to a reduction in the total time spent on recording.

Most of the plans, whatever their format, record variances to the standard plan of care for each patient (exception reporting). This can be an effective audit tool to examine clinical practice as it documents any variance (exception) to the expected plan of care, whether that is because the care was not given or because it was above the standard set in the plan. Analysis of the variances to care for a number of patients allows review as to the actual care being received by patients and can highlight any deficiencies in the system. It also clarifies what is actually happening in practice; this may not always match the professionals' assumptions. Variances usually identify anomalies in the system, which are simple to iron out, e.g. the fact that only a doctor can refer a patient for physiotherapy, thus delaying physio when the doctor forgets. The answer in a multidisciplinary care plan, is to agree the trigger factors for referral, to enable any health care professional to undertake the referral.

Monitoring of adverse events

An adverse event can be defined as an unexpected or undesirable occurrence during a health care episode which has, or has the potential for, a negative impact on a patient, resulting from some aspect of health care. A group of reported adverse patient incidents or events can be a useful tool for looking at clinical practice and reviewing it. The impetus may come from within one profession, but on closer examination may be found to involve several groups of the multidisciplinary team.

The aims of such an approach will include: producing reports and analyses which clinical staff will find useful, accurate, timely and meaningful; translating information on adverse events into changes in clinical practice and quality improvements when they are indicated; assessing the cost implications, both financial and diversion of resources away from other patients, of adverse events within the hospital. One example of this has been used at the Royal National Orthopaedic Hospital, Stanmore, through looking at a number of reported nursing drug administration errors. When these were examined in depth, several were found to be linked with unclear or incomplete drug prescriptions by the medical staff. As a result, a drug chart audit was carried out within one of the directorates over a 10-day period, involving nursing, medical and pharmacy staff. A total of 45.5 per cent of the patients in the audit had prescription errors on their charts. Of these, 80 per cent had more than one error noted. In addition, the average time taken by the medical staff to correct errors, once they had been notified of them, was 2 hours 20 minutes, with a range of 30 minutes to 9 hours 45 minutes.

Predominantly, the audit highlighted the fact that junior medical staff were not correctly prescribing drugs in accordance with hospital policy. Nursing staff were having to spend a great deal of time in contacting doctors to correct prescription charts, and particular difficulties arose when the patients' doctors were in the operating theatre.

These results were presented to both medical and clinical audit meetings and a number of recommendations were made, including an update on prescribing for all junior medical staff during their induction programme. It was also noted that the hospital drug chart was inappropriate for long-term patients who are in hospital for more than two weeks, so a group has been set up to devise a new drug chart more appropriate for the rehabilitation patient.

Clinical audit

While uniprofessional audit will continue to have an important role, the care of patients depends on the combined contributions of a number of professionals, so future approaches to audit need to reflect this.

Clinical audit, which takes a wide multidisciplinary approach, is the way forward but must be introduced in an evolutionary way. Davison (1990) argues that it would be unfortunate if the enforced inclusion of nursing staff and professions allied to medicine in the audit process was felt to be threatening to medical staff so that they 'refused to play'.

However, medical audit should not be allowed to become a 'secret society' which takes place behind closed doors. This is often justified by doctors on the basis of protecting patient confidentiality and the dangers of exposing themselves to potential litigation. Nursing and therapy audit is currently much more open in terms of its process and results. The Department of Health (1993) is quite clear that audit should only be confidential at the individual patient/clinician level. There is also a great deal of disparity at a national level in terms of the funding available to support medical audit (£41.9 million in 1993/94) and nursing and therapy audit (£8.2 million in 1993/94). This does not in any way facilitate collaboration on audit between the two groups and it has been successfully argued that the money should simply be distributed to support *clinical* audit. It is not easy to create the right culture in which open discussion and an honest review of performance can take place. Any review and self-criticism must be followed by action as there is no point in investing time and energy if a change of behaviour and/or practice does not result. This change is dependent on the multidisciplinary team's willingness to accept the part each member plays in delivering the service, and on the team's ability to work together to solve problems.

Medicine and nursing already perceive their traditional roles as threatened by each other due to such issues as the reduction in junior doctors' hours. The Department of Health is pressing hard for a number of the roles and responsibilities currently undertaken by junior doctors to be delegated to other health care professions, particularly nursing. Nursing, in return, feels that it may have little say in what is handed to them, but there is a real need for the professions to work together to provide the best solutions to the efficient delivery of patient care.

Teamwork

Nurses and therapists are often wary of being 'swallowed up' by their medical colleagues, who they feel are more powerful in terms of their status and support from the Department of Health, as reinforced by the disproportionate funding of audits. They also feel that only when they become more confident in auditing their own practice, will they be able to play an active role within clinical audit. In addition, doctors must accept the professional credibility of other members of the health care team. Nurses and therapists need to feel valued by their colleagues in order to expose themselves to audit. Historically, nursing has always been under scrutiny, initially from the medical profession and latterly from managers, and has often been subject to adverse criticism through such vehicles as skill-mix reviews. It is interesting to note that nearly all medical audit assistants are nurses. While it can be argued that health care knowledge is useful when supporting an audit process, does this in fact work to reinforce the handmaiden role of nurses to doctors?

The whole audit process, therefore, must be clinically owned and clinically led as it will not work if it is felt to be imposed from on high. To be worthwhile, it must be continuous, remain an ongoing and permanent feature and involve all activities and all staff. It is the business of everyone and must be supported and encouraged by managers. All health care professionals must work together to foster understanding and respect for the contribution each makes to patient care.

Firth-Cozens (1992) argues that effective team working is very different from old styles of organisational and managerial structures, which were based on a hierarchy with one person in overall charge. An effective team will welcome differing views, but at the same time work towards consensus and managing conflict.

Conflict within groups is inevitable. However, a team which is working effectively will enable its mentors to acknowledge the pressures and work out their differences. Individual defence mechanisms as a reaction to change can be dealt with by drawing attention to the reality of the difficulties as they apply to everyone and so give permission for fears rather than defences. Using an analytical approach such as this will require discussion and cooperation between the different health professionals, which will generate a better understanding of how others work and how that work contributes to patient care.

All this will take time to carry out. Time spent in audit will be lost to direct care of patients. Audit has been criticised for this, usually by people who do not want to be involved in it. However, the loss of clinical time must be seen in context. It could be argued that any busy clinician must set aside time to stand back and take a detached view about what he/she is doing and how well he/she is doing it (Davison, 1990). By taking time out, a better sense of proportion and of priorities and practices should be developed. Cessation of clinical work within the hospital, for example, closure of outpatients departments and operation theatres for a session, allows legitimate time to be set aside for audit within the working day, enables a wide group of professionals to attend and makes managerial support explicit. Normand (1992) identified one of the constraints in audit as a 'lack of legitimacy' for time to be devoted to the process. This can be seen in two ways: the need to actually find time, and the need to make it respectable to take time out of patient care and devote it to quality and audit.

Brian Edwards, in addressing the 1993 Clinical Audit Conference 'Measuring Quality', made the following points:

- Audit cannot be an optional extra – it must become an organisational and personal rock in the middle of clinical practice.
- There is a place for both uniprofessional and wider clinical audit, but the direction of travel must be the ability to audit an individual patient's total experience, including the non-clinical aspects of care.
- Clinical audit and the other features of quality assurance must grow closer and closer together. Shared data collection systems are part of the way forward.
- The NHS needs a more effective mechanism for sharing the results of the clinical audit process.
- The process of audit must always excite rather than threaten health care professionals. Mistakes are part of the learning process. We owe it to the community we serve to learn quickly how to serve them better.

Perhaps one of the main things which can emerge from a multi-professional approach to audit is more emphasis on the main objective of any health care, which is the quality of the outcome for the patient. Individual professions easily become focused on their own assessments and interventions. Bringing the professions together highlights the final outcome for the individual patient. Normand (1992) sees the greatest challenge of multi-professional audit as coming from the improved focus on whether people have really been helped to be independent. Good quality care and the best quality outcomes can only be achieved by working together.

Clinical audit, therefore, is very much concerned with what happens to the patient rather than what the various professionals involved in care do. Many units are now beginning to look at multidisciplinary treatment protocols which are addressed under a variety of titles, including collaborative care plans, care maps, critical paths and anticipated recovery paths (mentioned earlier in this chapter, and described in detail in Chapter 3). All these approaches have a number of goals in common:

- To standardise outcomes and cost of care.
- To promote collaborative practice between medical, nursing and paramedical staff.
- To determine the best mix of resources and methods to achieve clinical and patient satisfaction outcomes.
- To minimise variation in the clinical management process.

A number of benefits can also be identified from the process, including:

- Improved patient outcomes through a better understanding of which activities impact upon the outcome.
- Professional satisfaction of staff by linking their activities to identifiable patient outcomes.
- Movement towards change in clinical practice.
- Monitoring actual practice against the assumed norm.
- Teaching tool for junior staff.
- Enhanced awareness of the contribution of other professions.
- Increased patient involvement in care planning.

How do we set about initiating multidisciplinary audit? Perhaps most importantly, professionals need to be taught how to audit care together. Health care professionals do not instinctively know how to carry out audit and joint education could be one step towards breaking down the socialisation process that leads to unequal relationships within the care team. This educational process should incorporate the different perspectives of each professional's role in the cure–care continuum, to enable each professional to recognise the worth of the other, and thus to contribute to meaningful review of the service and practice.

McKenna (1992) comments on what he sees as a piecemeal approach to quality assurance in patient care, with nurses working in isolation to obtain confidence and doctors to retain independence. A situation where uniprofessional control is seen as more important than interprofessional communication may not only minimise the impact of any audit programme but also result in a poor service of poorer quality. Clifford (1985) argues that nurses and doctors work in the pursuit of quality care and goes on to say that:

> This quality of care will provide the only substantial rationale for any redefinition of boundaries between nursing and medical practice in the future.

The introduction of team working, based on the pursuit of quality care, into the audit process will make the achievement of better patient care a useful and worthwhile experience for all involved.

References

Audit Commission (1991) *The Virtue of Patients Making Best Use of Ward Resources*. London: HMSO.

Clifford C (1985) Nurse–doctor relationships: is there cause for concern? *Nursing Practice* **2**: 102–108.

Davison A J (1990) Action of audit. *International Journal of Health Care and Quality Assurance* **3** (6): 14–16.

Edwards B (1993) Keynote address, Measuring Quality. East Midlands Conference Centre, Nottingham.

Firth-Cozens J (1992) Building teams for effective audit. *Quality in Health Care* **1**: 252–255.

Keddy B, Jones Gilles M, Jacobs P, Burton H and Rogers M (1986) The doctor–nurse relationship: an historical perspective. *Journal of Advanced Nursing* **1** (1): 745–753.

Mackay L (1993) *Conflicts in Care: Medicine and Nursing*. London: Chapman & Hall.

McKenna H (1992) Quality quarantine: a call for less professional isolation. *Quality in Health Care* **1**: 215–216.

Normand C (1992) The challenge of a multiprofessional approach to clinical audit. Paper presented at Measuring Quality. East Midlands Conference Centre, Nottingham.

Simpson I H (1979) *From Student to Nurse*. London: Cambridge University Press.

Stein L (1967) The doctor–nurse game. *Archives in General Psychiatry* **16**: 699–703.

Surgeon K (1990) Managing in a professional bureaucracy. *International Journal of Health Care and Quality Assurance* **3** (2): 17–24.

White R (1988) *Political Issues in Nursing: Vol 3*. Chichester: John Wiley and Sons.

Wright S (1985) New nurses: new boundaries. *Nursing Practice* **1**: 32–39.

8

Audit and the Purchasing Process

Introduction

This chapter provides an overview of the purchasing function and describes key aspects of the role. To set purchasing of health care in a broader context, key aspects of the NHS reforms are described along with some of the challenges associated with undertaking health needs assessment and achieving health gain. The purchasing cycle is presented and the relationship between purchasers and providers explored. The different kinds of contract are described followed by brief consideration of the commissioner's role and interest in audit. The chapter does not attempt to address the specific issues relating to practice and audit but is written in the belief that the professions will make a significant contribution to developing the culture and systems in which audit and innovative practice will flourish.

The 1990 NHS and Community Care Act

The aim of the National Health Service is to secure continuing improvement in the health of the population by:

Adding years to life – an increase in life expectancy and reduction in premature death *and*

Adding life to years – increasing years lived free from ill-health, reducing or minimising the adverse effects of illness and disability, promoting healthy lifestyles, physical and social environments and, overall, improving quality of life (Department of Health, 1992).

All developed countries are struggling to find new ways of responding to profound challenges, including: an increasing number of older people who will inevitably require health care and support in their later years, ever escalating and expensive medical technology, burgeoning consumer expectations, years of high inflation and a deep economic recession. Finite resources must be applied to meet the potentially infinite need for health care. The 1990 NHS and Community Care Act has produced widespread change. It was designed to stimulate efficiency and quality by allowing market forces to influence the delivery of health care. Key aspects of the reforms involved:

Establishment of a purchaser–provider split In future, money would follow patients through contracts for services rather than simply be given to provider units on a routine annual basis. District health authorities would no longer be responsible for directly managing the delivery of health care. Instead they would be required to identify the health needs of their resident population and purchase services to meet those needs.

Creation of NHS Trusts These would, in principle, have greater management freedom than directly managed units and the scope for competing, along with other suppliers, for contracts in the 'internal market'.

Introduction of general practitioner fundholders (GPFHs) – who would be able to buy a limited range of services for their patients using money that would otherwise have been used by the district health authority for purchasing care.

Capital charges Before the reforms, buildings, expensive equipment and other assets were often regarded as a 'free good' and there were few incentives to ensure that managers made effective use of them. A technical financial mechanism was created by the reforms to ensure that in future providers of care would be 'charged' for the use of assets.

Medical audit DHAs and FHSAs should be responsible for overseeing the quality of medical care delivered to their population. Health circular HC(91)2 instructed purchasers to gain '*sufficient information to be satisfied about medical audit policies followed by provider units with whom they have contractual arrangements*'. Detailed guidance was provided by the Department of Health about how medical audit should be organised, for example, every doctor should participate, it was to be primarily an educational activity, professionally led, appropriately resourced and should provide managers with regular reports, anonymised to avoid identification of individual patients and doctors.

Although the enterprise culture now emerging in NHS Trusts is a relatively new feature, the fundamental role of providers of health care has *not* changed – they always were, and continue to be, expert in the management and delivery of services. Purchasing may be regarded as the *only* genuinely new feature of the reformed NHS. It is still in its infancy but those involved are steadily developing the systems and expertise needed to support this exciting new function.

Purchasing health care

A broad range of activities is undertaken to achieve improvements in the health status of a population. Health care, while making an important contribution, plays a relatively modest role in producing health *per se*. Freedom from war, a clean water supply, good housing, adequate nutrition and a safe environment are all of fundamental importance. If individuals also receive love and affection, a decent education and opportunities throughout life to develop their unique potential, they will be empowered to make informed health choices. Because health is profoundly affected by social, economic and environmental factors it is important to influence developments throughout society and to commission interventions designed to prevent illness and promote health. The purchasing agenda extends, therefore, beyond the mere contracting for health services.

District health authorities (DHAs), Family health services authorities (FHSAs) and general practitioner fundholders (GPFHs) all have responsibility for purchasing health care. Although their specific remits may differ there is a growing awareness that they must work together and, where possible, coordinate purchasing intentions. GPs have special knowledge about health and service provision. They help their patients make decisions about health options and, when necessary, enable them to access specialist care. GPs have an *agency relationship* with their patients by which they give information and translate the patient's expressed need into demand.

DHAs purchase all services on behalf of the non-funding GPs and the 80 per cent of services not yet included in the GP Fundholding scheme. FHSAs are increasingly involved in the purchasing of hospital and community services, they are also beginning to apply the principles of purchasing to primary care and they are producing health investment plans in conjunction with DHAs. The community care aspects of the reforms were implemented on 1 April 1993. Social services departments are now responsible for assessing the needs of individuals, producing a care plan and procuring the necessary services. Monies that were previously allocated by social security departments have been transferred to social services to enable them to purchase domiciliary services, day care, residential and nursing home provision. Each year they are required, in conjunction with DHAs and FHSAs, to produce a community care plan that describes the services available, recognising the contribution made by the voluntary and independent sectors.

The Health of the Nation

Published in July 1992, *The Health of the Nation* provides us with the first NHS strategy for health. Five key areas in which it is possible to achieve substantial and longer term improvement in health status were identified, namely:

Coronary heart disease and stroke
Cancers
Mental illness
HIV/AIDS and sexual health
Accidents

The strategy highlights the need to improve health, not simply *health care*, and acknowledges that today's health problems need to be tackled by a range of measures, including action to improve health and prevent illness, improvement in diagnosis, treatment and rehabilitation and environmental quality.

Some of the key points are summarised below:

- It is essential that there is an appropriate balance between prevention, treatment and rehabilitation, all of which should aim to improve the quality, as well as the quantity, of life.
- The strategy is about making the best use of the resources the nation, as a whole, devotes to health. Decisions about the use of resources for new initiatives, research and development and health monitoring should reflect the priorities identified in the strategy.
- In framing action within key areas, the needs of specific groups of people within the population must be considered, for example, the particular needs of children, women, elderly people and people in black and minority ethnic groups and certain socio-economic groups.
- The role of the health professionals − and indeed everyone who provides health care and related services − will be crucial to the success of the strategy. The development and adoption of agreed standards of good practice is particularly important. The recent developments in clinical audit are to be commended and should be built on. Leadership in the development of good practice lies primarily with the health professionals and, where appropriate, the voluntary sector. (Note that the agenda has now shifted away from the medical audit towards clinical audit.)
- The Government is keen to explore with professional, voluntary and other bodies, opportunities for development and dissemination of standards of good practice, especially where these are developed collaboratively. The Government's Chief Professional Officers will discuss with the health professionals how further development of standards of good practice and clinical protocols can be put forward.
- The continuing success of the NHS is in improving quality of care, reducing waiting times, and increasing efficiency and value for money. The challenge for the NHS is to establish a more direct link between

what it does and the results in terms of improved health both for individuals and the population more widely.

- Increasingly, NHS authorities' performance will be measured against the efficient use of resources, and working with others, to achieve improvements in the health of local people.
- Systems are required for monitoring and appraising the health of the population, research and the measurement of health outcomes.

The strategy for health establishes a framework for the development of health care and clearly sets the purchasing agenda. The importance of creating *healthy alliances* – partnerships between purchasers and providers of health care, statutory, voluntary and commercial agencies, service users and informal carers – is a recurring theme. The need to be sure that we not only do the right things, but do them properly is also a key feature of the strategy. Purchasers and providers are urged systematically to evaluate current patterns of care, stop doing things that are ineffective and only adopt new interventions that have been shown to be effective.

The points summarised above emphasise the central role of clinical audit. Practice must be research-based and rigorously scrutinised to enhance effectiveness. Protocols that guide practice and assist audit have a valuable role to play. Purchasers of health care will pursue these issues and will be keen to contract with providers who demonstrate a commitment to audit. The responsibility for adding years to life and life to years is, however, a shared one. Nurses, midwives, health visitors and therapists account for a considerable proportion of NHS expenditure, have a high level of contact with patients and should, therefore, make a significant contribution to enhancing the health of the nation.

Health gain strategies

There are differing views about what is meant by health gain. In the report from the Association for Public Health (1992) the following definition is offered:

> Health gain is the sum of benefits arising from the application of NHS resources to improving the health of the population and delivering quality healthcare to individuals.

It has been suggested that health gain represents the profit of the NHS but it is much more difficult to measure than money. Quality is also difficult to define because it can mean different things to different people. Purchasers recognise the importance of finding a balance between the various components of quality. Although a number of criteria may be selected those identified by Maxwell (1984) are frequently applied, namely:

Access   Individuals should be able to gain access to services when and where they need them.

Equity   This means fairness rather than equality and recognises that people need differing levels of care to reach the desired outcome. It addresses the way in which we target and prioritise our services in response to health need, taking care to address the health needs of minority groups and those who have difficulty in self-advocacy.

Appropriateness and relevance to need   An appropriate service is one that the population or individual actually needs.

Effectiveness   Services must achieve the intended benefits and outcomes.

Acceptability   The quality of communication, courtesy and comfort are all important. The consumer must feel important, confident and in control.

Cost-effectiveness and efficiency   If used efficiently, our resources can be spread more widely. Cost-effective care is highly ethical, the aim must be to achieve the required standard of service at the lowest cost. Economies of scale must be fully harnessed, for example, expensive specialist services should be procured from a central place when it would be wasteful to provide them on a number of sites. Where possible the resources currently devoted to ineffective provision must be withdrawn and reinvested in more fruitful services – all activity has an 'opportunity cost' in that the money used could have been spent on something else.

When writing specifications, purchasers pay close attention to these criteria with a view to establishing a satisfactory balance and procuring services capable of achieving optimal health gain. Overall, interventions should improve the health status of the *population* as well as that of individuals.

Health needs assessment

Health needs assessment is fundamental to the reformed NHS and will, increasingly, inform purchasing. A considerable amount has been written about 'need' and it is not possible to give a detailed review of the theoretical issues in this chapter. It is important, however, for practitioners to recognise the nature of the challenge because they will then be able to contribute to the process.

Bradshaw (1972) described a taxonomy of need:

Normative need   The definition of need derived from professional judgement.

Felt need   An individual's self-perceived needs.

Expressed need A felt need that is translated into a demand for services.

Comparative need The needs of one person compared with those of another.

Each of the above approaches has limitations and pitfalls. Confusion arises about whether we are assessing general need, the need for health or the need for health care. Need is further complicated in that it changes over time; purchasers usually focus on need defined as *the ability to benefit from health care*. This depends on the incidence and prevalence of the condition and the effectiveness of the services available to deal with it.

Needs assessment should be closely aligned to the purchasing process. It requires a considerable amount of information about *morbidity* as well as *mortality* because the NHS must enhance the quality of life for people who are sick as well as prevent premature death. In addition to gathering and examining information about the health needs of the *total* population served, it is also necessary to work in a bottom up way with GPs and the primary health care team, to share their knowledge of the practice and locality, give them additional information gleaned from the broader analysis and assist them in identifying local needs and priorities. This is clearly a massive task and one that is further complicated by the way in which demand and supply affect need.

Health economists have demonstrated the interaction between need, demand and supply. Gabbay and Stevens (1991) provide the following definitions:

Need – what people benefit from.
Demand – what people ask for.
Supply – what is provided.

They provide a very useful model of the way in which these factors influence each other. Their theories are explored in some detail below because they illustrate the complex interactions and also because they provide a valuable framework for audit.

Gabbay and Stevens suggest that all health care interventions will fall within the numbered fields (Figure 8.1). Need is a subjective concept, affected not only by cultural and ethical determinants but also by the prevailing professional views about a given condition and the current research agenda. Need is not fixed but open to interpretation and it changes over time. Not all of the need for health care is met and frequently those who need it most fail to access the relevant service. For example, there is considerable evidence that many women who are found to have cervical cancer have not had routine smear tests. This situation falls within field number 6 because there is need and supply but no demand. Field 1 deals with need for which there is neither supply nor demand, for example, health promotion clinics for homeless people.

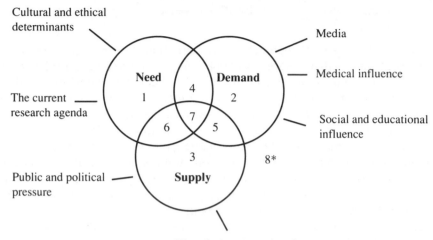

Figure 8.1 Need, demand and supply: influences and overlaps (Gabbay and Stevens, 1991)

Field 3 might include the performance of routine caesarean sections (on women who have had a previous section) which are neither demanded nor needed but continue to be supplied. Many nursing duties that for many years were undertaken in a ritualistic way, also fall within this field, such as four-hourly observations of temperature, pulse and blood pressure or the routine shaving and administration of enemata to women in labour.

Services that are demanded and supplied but not needed fall within field 5. The routine inspection of school children for head infection is an example of this. In this situation the *real* need is, arguably, for parents to be given the necessary knowledge and skills to enable them to perform the task with confidence.

Demand is influenced by many things including social and educational factors, the media and medical profession. Waiting lists for surgery describe demand, which may be influenced by supply, but which may or may not be needed. Utilisation rates describe supply that may be demanded, or needed, or both. For example, a health visitor may have a high client contact rate but this does not automatically mean that she is addressing need; some contacts may, for example, be the result of rigid historical visiting policies.

Gabbay and Stevens suggest that any useful assessment of needs will require not only an analysis of the relationship between need, demand and supply for many conditions under consideration but also an attempt to see how the three can be made more congruent. The goal should be systematically to expand field 7. This will clearly require considerable epidemiological research.

Purchasers expect that, in addition to contributing to research, practitioners will critically examine all aspects of care to consider whether they are meeting need, responding to demand or simply delivering services that follow an historical pattern of delivery without any sound justification. When analysing inputs such as staffing levels, clinical procedures, utilisation rates and outcomes, the interrelationship between supply, demand and need must be explored.

The purchasing agenda

In February 1993, Virginia Bottomley made the following statement:

> The key to developing the NHS internal market lies with health authorities and fundholders, the purchasers of care. They have five basic tasks: assessing the needs; setting the standards; targeting the resources; demanding value for money; and lastly, monitoring the quality . . . From first to last, it is the purchasers who could be in control. They pay the piper. They must call the tune . . . (Health Circular 93/575; DoH, 1993a)

A number of issues and initiatives help to shape the purchasing agenda, some of which are listed below:

- *Health of the Nation.*

- *The Patient's Charter* – with its emphasis on consumerism and waiting times.

- Public empowerment and consumer involvement in assessing health needs, identifying priorities and monitoring performance – because health and health care are value laden it is important to balance the professional and public perspectives.

- Increased emphasis on health promotion.

- Developing Primary Care, enhancing the interface between secondary and primary care and, where appropriate shifting services and resources to primary care.

- Development of 'healthy alliances'.

- Collaborative purchasing – working with GP Fundholders and Social Services to secure cost-effective and properly integrated provision and smooth implementation of Care in the Community. In addition, FHSAs are taking increased responsibility for managing GP Fundholding.

- Maintenance of a comprehensive supply of health care that is need rather than service led.

- Contract negotiation and monitoring.

- Priority setting through needs assessment.

The purchasing cycle

Figure 8.2 illustrates the purchasing cycle. As mentioned above, purchasing is still in its infancy. Great strides have been made in establishing a framework for undertaking health needs assessment, interpreting the findings, writing service specifications and contract negotiation. Further work is needed, however, on prioritising investment to secure maximum health gain, supplier selection, contract monitoring and service evaluation.

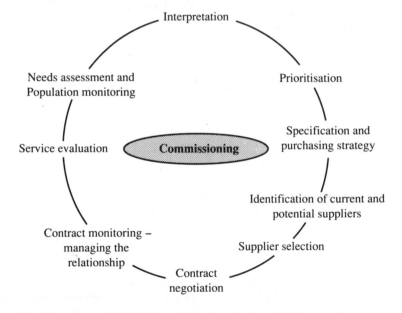

Figure 8.2 The purchasing cycle

Provider selection

Purchasing may be a relatively new concept in the NHS but there is a considerable amount of transferable expertise in the commercial sector. To a large extent, NHS purchasers have continued to use their historical suppliers for most of their requirements and have not as yet begun the process of rigorous supplier review with a view to making major shifts in contracts. The Institute of Purchasing and Supply recommends the comprehensive evaluation of potential suppliers and has produced a checklist of areas which warrant particular attention (Lysons, 1990):

a. Personal attitudes The attitudes of employees towards their work – this provides an indication of the likely quality of their output and service dependability. The state of morale will be evident from:
An atmosphere of harmony or dissatisfaction among staff
The degree of interest in customer service
The degree of energy displayed in getting things done
The use of manpower – whether economical or wasteful.

b. Adequacy and care of equipment Is it:
Modern or antiquated?
Accurately maintained or obviously worn?
Well cared for or neglected?
Of the right capacity and type?

c. Technological know-how Does the supplier have the required level and range of expertise?

d. Means of controlling quality Observations of the quality systems and inspection methods will indicate their adequacy.

e. Housekeeping A pleasant and clean environment indicates good management and inspires confidence that the same care will be given to its services/products. The dangers of breakdown, fire and other disasters will also be minimised.

All the above criteria can be applied to the selection of suppliers of health care. Attention should be given to the organisational structure to ensure that there are clear lines of responsibility and authority, sufficient staff with relevant skills, robust quality systems with documented procedures and standards, effective implementation, monitoring, reporting and change management. Evaluation of the organisational culture is equally important to ensure that it is value driven (by the right values), has strong leadership, integrity and capacity for change and innovation. A learning culture, one that demonstrates a high level of commitment to teamwork, education, training, audit, research and change, will be sought. It should also be highly responsive to the needs and expectations of consumers and purchasers.

The purchaser will wish to buy only those services that are effective. In addition to the criteria mentioned above, providers must be able to demonstrate the positive outcomes resulting from their work.

Contracts

Contract documentation seeks to make explicit the roles and responsibilities of purchasers and providers in meeting the health needs of the population served. Documentation usually comprises sections on each of the following:

The terms of the agreement
Service specifications
Quality requirements
Information requirements
Financial terms and agreed activity levels.

The service specification is of great significance and involves a considerable amount of work on the part of both purchaser and provider. Although they may be very brief the trend will be for them to specify key elements of clinical practice.

Purchasers of health care have a finite amount of money and must ensure that expenditure balances with the financial allocation and that providers achieve the agreed activity levels within recurrent financial resources. They are also frequently obliged to achieve efficiency savings. These may either produce *extra* activity for the same amount of money or the same amount of activity for *less* money, while at the same time enhancing effectiveness. Sometimes this may involve stopping ineffective work.

Provider units must earn *all* their income – failure to win contracts for services means they will have no money to deliver care or pay staff. They must deliver the specified services, maintain a break-even on expenditure and income and assure the quality of treatment and service. All staff have therefore a clear responsibility for making efficient use of resources and making a full contribution to promoting the future viability of their organisation.

Contracts with NHS providers are not legal documents. The NHS market is managed internally and any disputes are settled by arbitration. Contracts can range from being very general to very specific; the degree of sophistication depends on the quality of information available on which to set and monitor them, the nature of the service and also on the amount of financial risk the parties feel able to handle. A brief summary of the *main* types of contract is provided below:

Block   A contract which provides a defined range of services, with limited service volumes over a period of time for which the provider is paid an annual sum in instalments. The purchaser is basically buying a given level of capacity. These are very broad based and guarantee contract income for the provider. They can be unsatisfactory from the provider's perspective if activity levels or case mix are higher than expected. Similarly the purchaser could waste money by buying more capacity than was actually needed if activity was lower than anticipated. They do not offer sanctions or incentives and money does not follow individual patients.

Cost and volume   A contract in which the provider receives an agreed sum of money in return for treating a specified number of patients within minimum and maximum activity levels. These have more clearly defined service and volume specifications so need a more comprehensive assessment of health need. The purchaser may need to set aside some money as a contingency, in case activity is required to exceed the maximum level. Also, both parties must track patient treatment levels carefully. Financial risk is shared and the purchaser may include incentives and sanctions.

Cost per case   A contract in which the purchaser agrees the amount to be paid for the treatment of *individual* patients. These are very clearly specified 'one-off' deals which generate cash on delivery. Although they give the purchaser considerable scope for selecting the 'best' provider for the individual they also generate a massive amount of paperwork and high management costs for both parties – which can waste NHS resources. They do not give the provider any financial security and as such are unlikely to create a sense of long-term partnership. *Extra contractual referrals* (ECRs) are cost per case contracts. At the start of each financial year DHAs set aside a small percentage of their purchasing budget to pay for them. If the number is higher than expected or if the referrals are for very expensive care, such as forensic psychiatry, then the DHA will have difficulty balancing its books.

It is obviously important for providers to cost their services as accurately as possible. The Department of Health stipulates that:

Price must equal cost – they are not allowed to make a profit.

All providers should state their prices.

Prices should be worked out at full cost (marginal costing is only allowed where there is spare capacity for a short period).

There should be no planned cross-subsidisation between services.

Costs can be classified and attributed to activity in a number of different ways. It is important for senior nurses and therapists to understand how their services have been dealt with. It is not possible to provide further details in this chapter but an excellent, user-friendly description of financial issues can be found in the *Introductory Guide to NHS Finance*, published by the Healthcare Financial Management Association in 1991. Similarly, practitioners will wish to have a good working knowledge of resource management. *Using Information in Managing The Nursing Resource* (the 'rainbow pack') is highly recommended. (Published by North West Thames RHA in conjunction with Greenhalgh & Company Ltd.)

Contract monitoring must be undertaken by both the purchaser and provider. Failure to keep track of the activity carried out for each purchaser can result in the loss of income for providers, so accurate documentation is essential. Many providers are introducing sophisticated information systems that will support clinicians and general managers in decision making and provide high quality information on contract performance. Information also helps the purchaser to: determine health needs; monitor the relationship between demand and supply; monitor waiting lists; compare the performance of different suppliers; ensure that they comply with their contracts; give value for money. Ideally, contract monitoring information should be built into the operational systems of the provider units so that it is only collected and entered onto a computer once and subsequently used for management purposes by purchasers and providers.

Information is the lifeblood of complex organisations – it empowers people to make decisions and manage change. To be of value, it must be accurate, complete, relevant, timely and 'owned'. Unless it is credible it will not be properly used and if it is not used it will always be of poor quality. At present, much of the information routinely collected and reported to purchasers relates to activity and cost, but purchasers recognise that performance on quality is equally (if not more) important. It is relatively easy to monitor *quantitative* aspects of quality such as waiting times but much more difficult to capture information about *qualitative* dimensions. Purchasers and providers must be prepared to share relevant information because this will reduce the cost of obtaining it and promote cost-effectiveness.

The relationship between purchasers and providers

In the early days of the NHS reforms the new culture of competition appeared to produce some aggressive posturing on the part of both purchasers and providers. There was a tendency to equate survival in a competitive environment with a 'macho' style of management. There is now increasing evidence that all parties are beginning to adopt a more balanced, partnership approach. Now that the majority of provider units have become NHS Trusts, purchasers are able to focus more clearly on their new role and develop purchasing strategies. As indicated earlier, they are also reviewing sources of supply. For every aspect of provision this involves exploring a wide range of issues, including:

● The balance of provision between primary and secondary care – should there be a shift?

● The location of hospital care – how many places should deliver the service? In which geographical areas? Are there economies of scale that should be harnessed by centralising the source? Does the current provider perform satisfactorily? What preferences have been expressed by consumers and GPs?

● The ideal number of suppliers and the desired nature of the relationship, for example, short, medium or long term.

Some contracts can be switched more easily than others. For example, it may be feasible for the majority of patients to travel a reasonable distance for elective surgical treatment but not for emergency medical care and many aspects of mental health care. Purchasers are unlikely to want to chop and change suppliers frequently because this would reduce their scope for influencing the provider and getting 'added value' from the contract, lead to confusion for GPs and consumers and generate additional costs associated with managing the switch itself. In parts of the country, however, where there are currently too many units wanting to produce more care than is actually needed (i.e. over capacity) then clearly competition will be fierce and the providers that can offer the best deal will be rewarded. The best deal does not necessarily mean the cheapest; all of Maxwell's dimensions of quality must be considered, but if all else is equal then cost will be a powerful lever for change.

With the goal of producing optimal health gain for every pound spent, purchasers will naturally seek to exercise maximum leverage and drive down costs where these are higher than necessary due to poor management. Effective management involves setting ambitious but achievable targets and enabling constructive change. Contracts should be seen as a vehicle for change rather than as a mechanism for promoting conflict. There is ample evidence in the commercial sector of a shift away from ruthless competitive tendering towards what is frequently described as partnership sourcing.

Partnership purchasing is an arrangement between the purchaser and provider by which the two parties undertake to use their combined resources to better meet the needs of the consumer. It requires commitment to a long-term relationship, cooperation, trust, compatibility of cultures, the constant search for better solutions, time to develop, openness and communication, mutual benefit, excellent measurement systems and the perception of success (Griffiths, 1992). Partnership purchasing does not automatically result in single suppliers. A competitive process can be used to select suppliers and several may be chosen, however the nature of the relationship, including the commitment to investment in each others business, tends to reduce the number used. For many aspects of health care the collaborative (but not cosy) partnership approach has much to offer and it is reasonable to assume that the NHS will follow this trend once the market has 'shaken out' both excess supply and badly managed organisations. Meanwhile providers will wish to make sure that *they* are the preferred providers of the future.

The purchasers' role in audit

In February 1993 Dr Kenneth Calman, the Chief Medical Officer, announced that £51.6 million would be available for clinical audit in 1993/94. Stressing that everyone who works in the NHS has a professional duty to ensure the best possible quality of care and clinical outcome for their patients, he indicated the need to shift to team based audit, involving professionals and managers. With reference to the relationship between purchasers and providers he said:

> Audit has implications for purchasers and providers. In order to have confidence in the local audit programme, they must be part of it, that is, have an influence on the content of individual programmes and be assured that adequate action is being taken in response to audit findings (DOH, 1993b).

Mrs Moores, the Chief Nursing Officer, added:

> Although audit is important, it is only one tool in the achievement of continuous quality improvement in delivering patient care. Audit needs to be firmly embedded in the NHS management organisation. There is no room for complacency, Audit is everybody's business (DOH, 1993b).

These quotes succinctly summarise key challenges and potential sources of tension. The previous section considered ways in which relationships may evolve. The degree of intimacy will obviously be influenced by the *size* and complexity of the contract, its duration and geographical *proximity* of the provider to the purchaser. For example, if the purchaser negotiates a long-term contract with a local provider worth £5 million/year it is more likely that they will have a closer relationship than would be the case for a one-off contract worth £50,000 with a provider 100 miles away. In either case, the purchaser will have evaluated the organisation's 'fitness for purpose' before agreeing the contract and will have incorporated quality measures into the specification.

Purchasers are responsible for overseeing the quality of care delivered to their population. As a general principle they will focus on *'the what'* (i.e. specifying the outcome leaving the provider to address) *'the how'* (i.e. managing the inputs and processes in a way that delivers the desired outcome). Most purchasers will fulfil their obligation by monitoring the *systems* and *culture* of provider organisations rather than by interfering unnecessarily or trying to audit every detail themselves. Purchasers will expect providers to establish comprehensive quality structures, plans and systems and ensure that audit activity is built into everybody's work, including, for example: the ongoing audit of care undertaken by individual staff in conjunction with patients; peer review; audit of in-house and *Patient's Charter* standards; critical incidents; patient satisfaction; complaints; and focused audit of key indicators of quality, both within and across teams.

In addition to evaluating routine monitoring reports, the purchaser is likely to make monitoring visits to gain a greater understanding of the quality of care provided and make a qualitative assessment of certain aspects of quality. They will wish to ascertain the level of commitment to audit – the extent of involvement, professional leadership and ownership of the process, reports produced and action taken.

Clinical audit has a valuable role to play in demonstrating service effectiveness. It should address the structure, process and outcome of care. Outcome must be related to specific objectives and does not always mean cure. Negative outcomes often relate to disease, disability, distress and death.

Although purchasers will prefer to use outcome as the key measure of performance, for a variety of reasons it may be necessary for them to refer to measures of input and process. For example:

- When auditing a potential provider with a view to negotiating a contract with them.

- Where outcome measures are not available – for many services it is notoriously difficult to attribute outcomes to either inputs or processes. Practitioners may be confident of the value of their interventions but in the absence of research based evidence the purchaser is required to make a leap of faith in the belief that health gain will be derived from the investment.

- Where poor standards and a poor outcome may not be quickly identified by managers, clients or their advocates, in services provided for especially vulnerable groups such as people with learning disability, the very elderly and people suffering from mental illness.

- Where there is an agreed correlation between certain aspects of input or process and outcome, such as, the availability of nurses with an RSCN qualification.

- Where outcomes appear unsatisfactory and further investigation is called for – in these circumstances the purchaser may choose not to offer a subsequent contract, or, if the provider is the main source of supply in a long-term relationship the purchaser will be obliged to intervene to whatever extent necessary to resolve the problem.

There is a tendency for all organisations experiencing significant change to seek out what appears to be a magical solution, devote a great deal of energy to it for a short while, stimulate a modest amount of real commitment and a higher level of ritual dancing while reinforcing the small but deep seam of cynicism that plagues all sectors. The principles of total quality management (TQM) include a commitment to audit and undoubtedly have a great deal to offer but should not be seen as an automatic panacea or quick fix.

It is important to recognise that the culture of TQM is vastly different from that which has been prevalent in many parts of the NHS and that organisational culture cannot be changed quickly or easily. TQM and audit rely on teamwork, involvement, openness, a preparedness to celebrate small improvements, the constant search for quality improvements at the lowest cost and a bias to action.

Audit is central to professional practice, it requires intellectual curiosity, confidence, supportive systems and passion. It also requires trust and bravery – especially if conducted across different disciplines. Although there will always be some aspects of care that need a unidisciplinary audit, these are relatively rare. Audit can consume a considerable amount of time and, as such, is an expensive activity; there is an urgent need, therefore, to break down the barriers between different professions, between professionals and general managers and between purchasers and providers so that we can share information, knowledge and skills and work together to demonstrate the value of audit. An extraordinary amount of progress has already been made but there is no room for complacency. It requires a long-term commitment from purchasers and providers.

To facilitate this process it is the responsibility of each of us to create an open and supportive culture. While action must be taken to address deficits in practice, audit must not be seen primarily as a tool for searching out bad apples. Overload is also a major deterrent to innovation – it is much better to do a small amount of audit well than tackle a huge amount and do it badly. Audit must therefore be systematic rather than random, properly resourced and fully integrated into existing systems. It must be linked to continuing education and research and given high status, for example, by inviting teams to present their findings and action plans to Trust boards and incorporating them in quality reports to purchasers.

Purchasers will encourage the production of clinical protocols but will wish to avoid paying for unnecessary duplication. The Eli Lilly National Clinical Audit Centre, Leicester University, is making impressive headway in producing tried and tested protocols, which can be used nationally in primary care. This initiative will avoid the costly reinvention of numerous wheels and will be highly valued by practitioners and purchasers. Protocols must however be 'owned' by those who use them if change is to be generated. To date, relatively limited use has been made of performance indicators, largely due to the difficulty of comparing 'like with like'. In a tightly funded, competitive environment this situation will change. Purchasers and providers will increasingly have access to better information and greater incentives to compare performance between organisations; benchmarking will rapidly become a feature of the NHS.

Priorities for audit

In addition to the routine audit that is incorporated into the work of teams, each year the Department of Health allocates funds for special audit projects. It is likely that, in future, these will be given to purchasers so that they can negotiate their use with providers and devote them to priority issues. Priorities will generally fall within three categories:

Obligatory areas that take forward the corporate goals of the NHS   Some of these will have already been well researched, such as *Health of the Nation* goals. For others, national and local standards will be established, for example, *The Patient's Charter*.

Areas of local concern to purchasers and providers.   These are likely to relate to issues of efficiency and effectiveness and be patient-focused. They would include topics like the management of pain and prevention of pressure sores. Whoever suggested the topic would have to make its case for inclusion in the next year's audit contract. Many of the topics would need a multidisciplinary approach.

Areas that individual professions would like to audit relating to their practice. These would include areas of local and national concern and would often be unidisciplinary.

Thus, a programme for audit within a provider unit will be funded by the purchaser and negotiated with the provider. The amount of information to be shared will also be negotiated. In general, the purchaser will require detailed feedback on findings relating to the first two categories. For the third, aggregated information will usually be required and the provider may be invited to suggest amendments to the service specification that arise from their audit. This way audit will be able to influence purchasing and drive forward standards of care both within and outside their own organisation. The purchaser would obviously want to be confident that the audit cycle had been completed.

Conclusion

The NHS reforms have certainly created new incentives to improve services and drive down costs. Within this context clinical audit has a pivotal role. Purchasers and providers of health care have common goals. They aim to be health gain focused, resource-effective and people-centred. The NHS needs a comprehensive range of viable providers who employ highly motivated staff and make a commitment to continuous improvement. Nurses and therapists have an important contribution to make to the identification of health needs, the development of service specifications that genuinely reflect best practice and to the creation of cultures and systems that support clinical audit. The NHS is publicly funded and sustained by the deep commitment of its employees, all of whom are accountable for the work they do. Purchasers and providers have specific roles but they must work together on many initiatives for the benefit of those served.

Clinical audit is definitely here to stay but to demonstrate its value it must be properly integrated into the work of individuals and organisations. Consumers also have an important role to play in audit and a systematic approach must be adopted to avoid creating 'survey fatigue'.

Purchasers and providers must strive to create learning organisations, minimise bureaucracy and duplication and maximise innovation, creativity and action. Quality must be built into every aspect of care, because no amount of monitoring will 'bolt it on' satisfactorily. The internal market has stimulated a welcome drive for cost-effectiveness but the question of what proportion of our nation's wealth should be devoted to health care is, and will continue to be, important. This will be determined by societal values and articulated through the political process. Meanwhile, it is the duty of each of us, while participating in this debate, to examine rigorously clinical practice to ensure that those services we do provide are cost effective and produce optimum health gain. Clinical audit is a valuable process and the shared responsibility of both commissioners and providers of health care.

References

Bradshaw J A (1972) In McLochlan J (ed.) *A Taxonomy of Social Need. Problems and Progress in Medical Care*. Oxford: Oxford University Press.

Department of Health (1992) *A Strategy For Health in England*. London: HMSO.

Department of Health (1993a) Health Circular 93/575, Press Release, 23 February.

Department of Health (1993b) Health Circular 93/553 Press Release, 11 February.

Gabbay J and Stevens A (1991) Needs assessment. *Health Trends* 23: 1.

Griffiths F (1992) Alliance partnership sourcing – a major tool for strategic procurement. *Purchasing and Supply Management*, May: 35–40.

Lysons C K (1990) *Purchasing*, 2nd Edn. London: M & E Handbooks.

Maxwell R S (1984) Quality assessment in health care. *British Medical Journal* **288**: 1470–1472.

The Association for Public Health (1992) Healthgain 1992 The Standing Conference – Gaining Momentum.

9

The Future for Audit

'Quality' and 'consumer responsiveness' sit alongside a fierce and continuing concern with economy and efficiency. It is not clear which group of values will take priority when (as at some point is inevitable) a trade-off has to be made. (Pollitt, 1993)

Such is the climate in which clinical audit is being championed by the NHS Management Executive (NHS ME). This dichotomy of values sums up the very heart of the difficulties that face all levels of the NHS in relation to the implementation of clinical audit. The key question has always been, and continues to be, how much resource do we as a nation spend on health care and what aspects of health care reap the best returns? However we may choose to view clinical audit, be it as a means to improve quality, a means to educate staff, or a means to reduce expenditure, we come back to the same issues of resource prioritisation and the development of new ways of working to meet the increasing demands of an ageing population, the new possibilities demonstrated by medical technology advances, and the increasing expectations of our consumers.

Within this book I have attempted to draw on the history of performance measurement to demonstrate that, while audit may possess some of the solutions to these issues, the issues themselves have been around a long time. Audit is one in a line of approaches to try and make sense of the concept of value for money as it applies to health care. As such we should therefore refrain from viewing it as an end in itself and should certainly make every effort to learn the lessons of the past by integrating audit into the very core of health care management and delivery, rather than treating it as an add-on 'luxury' for those that have the time. This in itself already causes us some difficulties. In order to introduce audit, the carrot of separate (and significant) funding alongside freedom to reduce clinical sessions, was dangled in front of our medical colleagues – a reasonably successful gambit aimed at encouraging them to adopt audit as their own. While being expedient at the time, this approach has now sent audit on a road that could lead to nowhere. We have seen from the chapters in this book, that in order for audit to contribute to real improvements in client treatment and care it must:

- Be multidisciplinary, based on partnership and mutual respect.
- Be undertaken within the context of the organisation in which solutions have to be found.
- Actively engage consumers in the process.
- Bridge the purchaser/provider split.
- Be part of a wider strategic approach to quality.
- Have demonstrable interfaces with research and with resource management.
- Be integral to the work of all professionals.
- Achieve changes in practices.
- Be owned at all levels of the organisation.
- Not be punitive, but rather be seen as developmental.
- Address local and national priorities in the name of public accountability.

Audit to date has rarely demonstrated success in any of these areas. To do so it requires a different track from the route taken so far by medical audit. This is not necessarily a backtracking, as the approach to medical audit has managed to involve some clinicians who would otherwise have resisted any form of scrutiny of their practice. It does require lessons to be learnt from the medical audit experience, many of which were taken on board by nursing and therapy audit, which has tended to concentrate more fully on multidisciplinary working, and on achievement of change. This reflection on past experiences will lead, in some cases, to the dismantling of structures put in place to support medical audit as a separate initiative, and reconfiguring clinical audit as an integral part of the hospital and community's work. It is always easy to look back with the benefit of hindsight and see how it could have been better achieved. The challenge now is to look forward to find a way of developing clinical audit that can really improve both client treatment and care, and staff satisfaction with their work, while maximising the resources available to achieve these ends.

National standards

The integration of audit into contracts is moving on apace with the instigation of work to develop national standards for good practice. These standards will form part of the contracting process. The work is seeking to draw on protocols already developed for medical, nursing and therapy treatment/care, within local settings, to develop guidelines for good practice that stand up to national scrutiny. Standards will reflect the current state of the literature in that field and will be the basis for negotiation between purchasers and providers within contracts. Subjects will be varied and will range from the medical model (e.g. inguinal hernia repair), to disease specific (e.g. asthma treatment), to the universal (e.g. pressure sore prevalence or wound management). In developing the guidance, it seeks to build on the initiatives being taken from within the service, e.g. protocol development; collaborative care plans; critical paths; care maps, to develop standardised descriptions of the care process and anticipated outcomes of that process. From these it should be possible to demonstrate those processes that achieve the best outcomes with the best use of resources.

While the attraction to develop national standards is an inevitable continuum from the work in auditing local standards, there will never be a definitive answer. As discussed in previous chapters, so much of a team's ability to deliver the best for clients is dependent on the culture of the organisation and the relative priority of that particular standard at that time. Moreover, it is always easier to develop standardised processes for uncomplicated procedures and clinical conditions than it is for more complex pathology. It is vital that we do not fall into the trap of making that which is easily measurable the priority for health care, to the neglect of the more complicated (therefore usually more vulnerable) clients that face us every day. As you can see from the examples above, it is often easier to describe standardised approaches for surgical conditions than for psychiatric conditions.

There is also the context of the research base to treatments and care; treatment receives significantly more funding through the clinical trials approach, than the 'softer' elements of care. We may well find that the psychosocial context in which treatment is delivered has more bearing on outcomes than the treatment itself. Thus, any development of national standards, while being welcomed, must recognise the differential status of the research base to nursing, therapy and medical professions and their domains of practice as well as the crucial contribution of the organisational culture in which care and treatment is delivered.

Whither committees?

To date, the distribution of funding for audit has been an add-on to baseline resources for any hospital or community service. Medical audit funding has been managed by a committee structure at both purchaser and provider levels. These committees review proposals for funding and prioritise them. They have been responsible for the annual audit report to the regional health authority (RHA) which was charged with managing the financial allocation. The RHAs sought to set up medical audit and manage the process of its introduction. Nursing and therapy audit has been managed in more diverse ways, from project funding to the funding of posts to develop a framework for audit. As we move towards clinical audit, the tendency is to create clinical audit committees that manage it, allocating

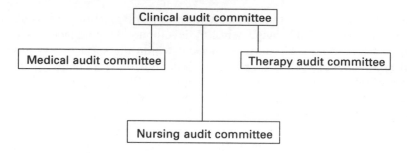

Figure 9.1 The committee quagmire

resources to profession-specific audits through sub-committees for medicine, nursing and therapists (Figure 9.1). This is directly as a response to medicine's fears that medical audit will lose out to multidisciplinary audit. These committees have varied terms of reference but tend to concentrate on resource allocation and monitoring. The clinical audit committee is usually dominated by doctors with token representation for nurses, managers and therapists. In order to represent all facets of medicine (which reflects the view that each specialty and consultant is autonomous in its practice), the committees are usually large and unwieldy. Such structures fail to capture the spirit of clinical audit as a fundamental part of the organisation's approach to quality, which must be everyone's business. The arguments to maintain the structure relate to the concept of audit as an add-on to clinical practice, requiring additional resources and the necessity to be accountable for these vast sums of money. The resources to support medical audit have been largely channelled into medical audit departments, and thus the committee structure seeks to manage the work of that department.

If clinical audit is to be fully integrated into the provider unit's work as part of the quality strategy and through the contractual process with purchasers, then the committee structure becomes redundant. As purchasers are charged with managing the financial allocation for clinical audit, they may seek to fund audit based on sets of priorities mutually agreed with providers; or providers may add on the costs of audit by case to the contract (see Chapter 8). Whichever method is chosen (and a mixture of the two is likely to emerge), priorities for audit will fall out of this negotiation process and accountability for the resources will be through the usual contractual lines. The work of the audit department will thus be planned for the year, based on these contracts, and the clinical audit process will move out from under the wings of the professionals to become a full part of service delivery. This does not negate the opportunity for profession-specific audit, rather it recognises that this will become an increasingly small part of audit activity as a whole.

Clinical audit departments

As with all initiatives that have been pump-primed from the centre, separate funding generates separate structures and support services. Hence the rise in the resource management department, the quality department and, more recently, the audit department. These departments are usually charged with some strategic work to develop the direction for the provider unit and with implementation of that strategy. The difference with the medical audit department has been the general lack of strategic work being undertaken. The department primarily responds to the requirements of the committees or individual professionals to produce audit reports through data collection and analysis, and to aggregate these into an annual report of total audit activity. As the employees within the department come from a range of backgrounds, this is usually the extent of their involvement and they have little authority for the completion of the audit cycle, i.e. the change process that is required as a result of the collection and presentation of data. The change management is left to the professionals undertaking the audit and being audited. This is an astounding weakness in the cycle (see section on change management in Chapter 2). While data collection and analysis is a vital part of the audit cycle, it becomes redundant if the professionals are unwilling or unable to change.

The instigation of audit through the contracting process will undoubtedly address this issue as audit areas are prioritised and actions will be expected by purchasers. The potential of audit departments is unrealised; there is real opportunity for strategic thinking to take place within these departments in order to present the provider's case for audit funding to the purchaser. It could become the pivotal point for prioritisation of audit activity and for internal monitoring. The expertise within the department could be used to educate all professionals in the audit process. If the audit department is to follow this path of strategy development, education, and monitoring, it requires management from within the general management structure. Moreover, the skills of audit assistants will then be recognised and career opportunities in other fields of project work or general management will open up. Undoubtedly, there will always be a role for data capture and analysis but this must take place within a framework for clinical audit agreed at Trust board level. It must be responsive to the interests and requirements of the NHS management executive, public opinion and expectations, professional's concerns, and the Trust's objectives within the business plan.

Consumer involvement

The greatest challenge to the professions may not be the exposure of audit within the contracting process, but the necessity to involve clients in audit.

The easy option is to involve them as passive recipients of our question-naires. The more difficult option is to involve clients in the prioritisation for selecting areas for audit and in the actual scrutiny of audit results. Initially, it could be seen that involvement will come from representative consumer groups. However, this does not recognise the changing nature of the contracting process, with the impetus towards much more patient focused contracts. There is a notion that every patient should be treated as if they were an Extra Contractual Referral (ECR), i.e. their care scrutinised by purchasers to ensure that they are getting the best value for money. If we are to develop more personalised contracting, with the associated case-specific monitoring, then the audit of individual cases against agreed protocols will be inevitable. If we are to adopt the thrust of patient-focused care, and empowerment, then patients' involvement in monitoring and assessing their own experiences will be fundamental. It will also mean that patients will have to be involved in drawing up the protocols against which they are being treated. This sounds like a marathon task and will undoubtedly involve a vast cultural shift from passive and uninterested consumerism to active involvement. The prime difficulty in such involve-ment is in the very nature of resource allocation.

Empowerment (i.e. choice) implies that there are choices to be made and that the best can be offered. We only have to open the newspapers to see that choice for some is already limited, as children fly to the USA to receive treatment funded from charitable donations or doctors restrict operating lists to the more healthy non-smokers. The quest for putting resource decisions into the public domain continues but it requires the public to accept the responsibility for those decisions, and as yet there are few signs that it is willing to do so. Whatever approach is taken, it must be followed with an understanding of the end-point and should address the issues of patient choice and the primacy of the patients' wishes. Ironically, it could be said that this is all icing on the cake, unless consumers are actually able to make choices about where and when they are treated, rather than relying on the surrogates of the purchasing authority or the GP fundholder. At minimum, patients should be able to question those purchasing health care on their behalf about the quality of that care and the benefits and drawbacks of receiving that care from a particular provider. This information must include audit results as indicators of clinical quality. The next challenge will be to make individual clinical staff accountable for their own clinical practice in such a public domain – something the professions have shirked for a very long time.

Information technology

Undoubtedly the future for audit is inextricably bound to the ability of information technology to respond to its requirements. If we are to audit each and every patient's experiences of the care process, then we will require patient-focused information systems that are able to provide relevant information quickly. The experiences within the NHS to date, demonstrate how very far we are from that ideal. It also requires us to be able to define and anticipate standardised patterns of care for all patients. The reality is that we will be lucky if we can accurately describe standardised patterns or protocols for as many as 60 per cent of in-patients. This means that the other 40 per cent will require individualised tracking mechanisms. Given that many hospitals have developed only one or two protocols to date, we can see that the achievement of this end is some way off. Moreover, as yet, the language for developing these systems is not available; although there are codes for medical diagnosis, these are not sensitive to nursing workload. A gentleman who has had a myocardial infarction will undergo a standard medical treatment pattern based on the specific diagnosis; however, the nursing care may be quite different for each patient, depending on that patient's home circumstances and physical and mental abilities. While medical diagnosis may be central for reasons of expediency, it does not address the full range of contributions to the client's health care.

Teamworking

Teamwork is emerging as the neglected but most vital element for successful clinical audit. Without effective partnerships and mutual respect, clinical audit will never address the actual problems facing patients and professionals. In order to undertake clinical audit, teams must have shared goals and objectives and must be committed to working together, rather than in tangent to each other. This requires an honesty and recognition of the rights of all parties to be involved on a par with each other, a factor that is not common, particularly within acute units. It requires the professions to recognise and turn their backs on the game playing of the past and to look for ways of building bridges and actively engaging on each other's 'territory'. All professionals taking part in audit will need to recognise and affirm the interdependence of their work. Polarisation of medicine as 'cure' and the other professionals as 'care' is unhelpful and inappropriate. In reality, the care–cure continuum is the playing field for all health care workers, with no profession having a right to monopolise one corner or put up 'no entry' signs. In order to bridge this gap, and to recognise it as a fundamental hindrance to the development of clinical audit, partnerships must be developed at the very heart of the professions – education. Until education is delivered on core subjects to all professions alike, and until those who educate are able to respect the contribution of all professions, then we face an uphill task. In addition, until research funding is allocated in recognition of the parity of professional contributions, those professions embarking on clinical audit without a secure research base to their practice will undoubtedly remain the underdogs. Any clinical audit strategy must address the issue of team building.

The next reorganisation!

It is difficult to know if clinical staff will notice any changes resulting from the most recent shake-up of the NHS bureaucracy, namely, the review of the intermediate tier. Undoubtedly, with clinical staff feeling the brunt of the 'vacancy factor', they will welcome any attempts to reduce the management overheads of the NHS. Many agree that, rather than a new reorganisation of the Service, this is just the logical completion of the ethos of *Working for Patients*, as the NHS management executive, and the regional health authorities had remained relatively unscathed by the fundamental changes which enabled the development of purchasing and Trusts. The bringing together of purchasing authorities to make larger, merged commissioning bodies, and then the integration of family health service authorities with these larger commissioning authorities, begins to feel like the re-emergence of the old area health authorities. This is further supported by the rapid reduction in the functions of the regions, with comparable reductions in the workforce at that level. This will inevitably push planning further down the organisation. The functions remaining at 'intermediate' level will inevitably be finance and general management in relation to the development and monitoring of commissioning. Professional functions such as public health are likely to be hived off to agencies which will be called on to provide advice as required. Political hot potatoes such as research and development will, for the time being, remain at intermediate level.

This reorganisation of the 'centre' signals a new approach to audit. Previously the development of audit was directed closely from the NHS ME, with regions taking a strong hand in its management. With a leaner and meaner central machine, it is likely that central control and dominance will have to fade, meaning that commissioners and providers will be forging the future for audit. The clinical outcomes group will remain to give broad direction and to provide the interface to government, but the responsibility for the interpretation of policy and its implementation will lie much further down the ladder than before. While all this will be welcomed by providers and professionals, it could come as a nasty shock to already overburdened commissioners, who were planning to wade into audit gradually, testing the water, rather than being plunged right in the deep end. All this is happening at a time when the auditors (in the form of the National Audit Office) are hot on the trail of the national audit programme, which has swallowed vast quantities of public money with questionable returns. Commissioners will rapidly need to develop the expertise and resources necessary to plan their strategies for audit, in order to reshape the audit agenda. If they do not do so now, the dominant professions within provider units will expand their current approach to medical audit into clinical audit, with all the pitfalls and wastage that currently exists. Audit committees will be here to stay.

Where next?

Clinical audit is emerging in very diverse forms, despite being centrally driven and led for some time. Diversity is taking the form of different methodologies for audit; the reliance on, and development of, IT; the relationship with other strategies within the Trusts; the 'openness' of audit; the involvement of consumers; the amount of cross-boundary inter-disciplinary collaboration; the involvement of managers and commissioners; the structures for audit; investment in audit; and the relative development of audit in acute and primary care settings. As with all that is new, the temptation is to seek the 'cookbook' approach, that is the recipe for success. And, as with all such initiatives, there are individuals and Trusts seeking to be the flagships and gurus for the 'only way' to make audit successful (i.e. make themselves successful). It is up to all those involved in audit to seek their own approach from the diversity that surrounds them, with particular reference to the situations facing providers and receivers of health care locally.

In this book I have attempted to dispel the myth that all you have to do is measure the 'current' against the perception of the 'best' to undertake meaningful audit. For many this will be a disappointment but in order actually to make something of audit, it is crucial that we face up to the realities of our patterns of working and behaviour and that we take the trouble to understand the nature of the organisation in which we work, and the undoubtedly difficult political arena in which we try and deliver a public service. Without at least some understanding of these issues, we will forever be disappointed and will be forever judged as unsuccessful. A Trust chairman once commented that audit had the potential to bring about more fundamental and lasting change than the NHS reforms could ever achieve. This comment showed great insight into the potential for audit and great understanding of the obstacles that stand in the way. There is real enthusiasm among many clinical staff to demonstrate the value of what they achieve on a daily basis and their worth to the NHS. This enthusiasm for, and commitment to, ever higher standards of care must be matched by the enthusiasm from the leaders of the NHS to provide sensible strategic goals for audit, as part of the wider remit of service development. Without the marrying of the two, clinical staff will become despondent and senior managers will become ever more alienated from clinical practice and professional judgements.

As with all things new, blame for lack of progress lies scattered along the paths of all health care professionals. There is always a tendency to be judgemental from a position of righteousness. In order for the efforts we have invested in audit to come to fruition, we need to take time to reflect on where we have come from and the challenges that face us over the next decade; we must then agree to bury the professional hatchets. This will not be easy, and to some it will smack of inaction in the face of adversity. However, without this gentle reflection and commitment to working together, the future for clinical audit looks set to go the way of all one-off, stand-alone strategies – mediocrity. In order to achieve fundamental improvements in care and to increase staff satisfaction, clinical audit must take on board the considerations listed in the first paragraph of this final chapter. Commitment to change and responsibility for personal practice is the order of the day.

Reference

Pollitt C (1993) *Managerialism and the Public Services*. 2nd Edn, p 189. Oxford: Blackwell.

Appendix 1 Staff Satisfaction Questionnaire

Introduction

Dear Colleague

Enclosed is a questionnaire on your feelings about your job. It is anonymous and therefore you will not be identifiable to myself or in the final study report. When completed, please seal the questionnaire in the envelope provided and return it to me

by

Thank you for your help

Instructions for completion

The questionnaire is in three sections. Please complete all three.

Section one:

The first part of the questionnaire asks for a list of things you find satisfying, and a list of things you find unsatisfying, about working on the ward.

Section two:

The second part consists of statements, each statement is accompanied by a scale that indicates a range of satisfaction. Please consider the statements, and mark with a tick, the box that is closest to your feelings. For instance.

A	B	C	D	E	F
Extremely unsatisfied	Very unsatisfied	Unsatisfied	Satisfied	Very satisfied	Extremely satisfied

	A	B	C	D	E	F
1. The opportunity to give total patient care.		✔				
2. Feeling that you are doing a good job.				✔		

I have indicated that I am very unsatisfied with the opportunity to give total patient care on the ward, and that I am satisfied with the feeling that I am doing a good job!

Section three:

The final section is for you to comment in more detail on any of the statements in Section 2. For instance, I may want to say that the reason for my dissatisfaction in the first statement above, is that I am never allocated the same patients.

Section One

Please list the 10 things that you think are most satisfying about working on the ward, in order of priority, starting with the most important, and ending with the least:

1.

2.

3.

4.

5.

6.

7.

8.

9.

10.

Please list the things you think are most unsatisfying about working on the ward, in order of priority, starting with the most important, and ending with the least:

1.

2.

3.

4.

5.

6.

7.

8.

9.

10.

Please go on to complete Section Two

Section Two

A	B	C	D	E	F
Extremely unsatisfied	Very unsatisfied	Unsatisfied	Satisfied	Very satisfied	Extremely satisfied

Working conditions
How satisfied/unsatisfied are you with:

	A	B	C	D	E	F
1. The working conditions on the ward, such as the environment and health and safety						
2. The opportunity to have variety in your work						
3. The work-load on the ward.						
4. The helpfulness of other staff						
5. The way you feel part of the team effort						
6. The physical surroundings provided for your patients						
7. The amount of work that can be realistically done						
8. The way the hospital treats its employees						
9. The adequacy of supplies, linen, utensils, nourishment for your patients						
10. The number of times you are required to cover for other wards						
11. The number of times your co-workers are sent to another ward						
12. The number of times you work overtime						
13. The amount of pay for the work you do						
14. Your Grade in relation to the work you do						

Emotional climate

	A	B	C	D	E	F
1. The opportunity to give total patient care						
2. The variety of tasks you are expected to perform						
3. The opportunity to perform the kind of tasks you do best						
4. The spirit of co-operation amongst your co-workers						
5. The way you are congratulated for good performance						
6. The opportunity to try new ideas						
7. The opportunity to perform duties for which you are best suited						
8. The opportunity to make decisions of your own						
9. The way you get credit for what you do						
10. The way the workload is shared						
11. The morale of other workers on the ward						
12. The opportunity to develop new and better ways of doing things						
13. The consideration given to your off-duty requests						
14. The pressure under which you work						

General

How satisfied/unsatisfied are you with:

	A	B	C	D	E	F
1. Your self-esteem or self-respect						
2. Practical guidance from other staff						
3. The opportunity for independent thought						
4. The opportunity for expression of doubts						
5. The feeling that you are doing a good job						
6. The opportunity to do challenging work						
7. Your interest in your work						
8. The opportunity for rewards from work						
9. Seeing effects of your personal contribution						
10. The opportunity to express your ideas						
11. The opportunity to develop your ideas						
12. The opportunity for useful learning on the job						
13. Generally speaking how satisfied are you with your job						

Please go on to the last section

Section 3

Please write below any comments you have about your responses to the questions in the previous section.

Appendix 2   Patient Telephone Survey

Introductory letter

Dear

I am conducting a survey on behalf of .... hospital, to try and find out what our patients think about the care they receive on the wards. I understand that you have recently been discharged from .... ward and would like to ask you a few questions about how you were cared for on the ward. To do this I would like to telephone you at your home next week. Your answers will be anonymised in the results of the survey, and will be completely confidential. Your cooperation would be most useful, as it will enable us to improve the service we offer, however you are under no obligation to take part.

I do hope that you will be able to give me your comments, both good and bad. I look forward to talking to you soon.

Yours sincerely,

Patient telephone interview schedule

Name: Other information:
Age:
Sex:
Operation/Investigation recorded as:

1. Could you tell me how long you spent on .... Ward?
    No prompts, this is just an introductory question.

2. I'm interested in finding out how you found things in hospital. Would you like to tell me how they took care of you on .... Ward?
    Prompts: the environment, the staff. What did you feel like? Was that what you expected? What do you mean by that? What sort of things are you referring to?

3. Could you name a nurse whom you found particularly helpful?

4. Why did you find that nurse helpful? *or* Can you remember what you did find helpful about the nurses?
    Prompt: Can you explain a little more for me? Why was that? What was helpful about that?

5. Did anything happen to you during your stay on .... Ward that upset or bothered you?
    Prompt: environment, staff. Why was that? What was it about that that upset/ bothered you? Did you complain about that?

6. Do you know what the operation/investigation was that you had?

7. Do you know what was wrong with you?

8. What instructions were you given about your health?
    Prompt: illness, looking after yourself.

9. Did you have enough information to look after yourself when you left hospital?
    Prompt: what information would you have liked?

Appendix 3   Collaborative Care Plan: Cholecystectomy*

Burton Hospital NHS Trust

Outcome goals

All patients will have attended a pre-admission screening clinic and given an admission date

By discharge the patient will display minimal or no signs of potential complications:
pain, cellulitis, bruising around wound, chest problems, leg problems
and will be ready for discharge on the third post-operative day

By discharge the patient/family will be fully conversant with the care plan and will have the opportunity to discuss with the multi-disciplinary team as appropriate:
the surgery and possible risks, prior to theatre
wound healing, possible complications and actions to take pain relief
diet modifications

By discharge physical and psychological needs will be met

* From: *Collaborative Care Planning – A Natural Catalyst for Change.* West Midlands Health Region Resource Management Support Unit. April 1991.

Day	Medical	Nursing	Dietician	Physiotherapy	Theatre	District/SW
Pre-Admission Clinic Date Signature	1) History and Examination 2) Assessment of risk factors 3) Arrangements for discharge 4) FBC/U & E 5) CXR 6) ECG 7) Allocate admission date	1) Urine test 2) Record weight and height 3) Discuss worries and problems 4) Start Kardex 5) Nurse contact telephone no. 6) Show patient ward 7) Visiting times				1) Assess suitability for early discharge 2) Assess the extent of social services and home nursing back-up required 3) Initiate arrangements for back-up as required
Pre-op Admission Day Date Signature	1) Assessment 2) Theatre list 3) Refer to Anaesthetist 4) Explain operation and consent forms 5) Medication *Heparin *T.E.D.S. *Prophylaxia *Antibiotics *Pre-medication *Sedatives	1) Welcome to ward – introduction to staff & patients 2) Baseline observations 3) Complete Kardex 4) Confirm social circumstances and discharge arrangements 5) Pre-operative talk 6) Skin preparation if necessary 7) Fast from . . . . 8) Safe custody of valuables	Low fat diet for lunch & evening meal	1) Introduction 2) Explain physiotherapy role 3) History – Assess mobility and listen to chest 4) Teach breathing and circulatory exercises and demonstrate supported coughing	Pre-op visit	1) If suitable for early discharge give notice to district nurse

Day	Medical	Nursing	Dietician	Physiotherapy	Theatre	District/SW
Pre-Admission Clinic Date Signature	1) Operation Notes 2) I.V. Rota 3) Analgesia	1) Bath and toilet 2) Check notes 3) Theatre check-list procedure 4) Check airway, position vital signs 5) Monitor pain – analgesia 6) Check wound and drain 7) Care I.V.I. 8) Wash hands and face 9) Sit up in bed 10) Breathing exercises		Remind post-op exercises		
First post-op Day Date Signature	1) check chest, legs, wound, drain 2) Assess fluids 3) Review analgesia 4) Discuss operation with patient and relatives	1) Analgesia 2) Bed Bath 3) Mobilize 4) Care of I.V.I. 5) Elimination 6) Check wound RVAC 7) 4-hourly TPR		Breathing & circulation exercises	Post-op visit	

Day	Medical	Nursing	Dietician	Physiotherapy	Theatre	District/SW
Second post-op day Date Signature	1) RVAC out if still in 2) Review analgesia 3) Check wound, neck, chest, legs	1) Discuss plan of care with patient 2) Mobilize for bath 3) Check wound 4) Light diet 5) 4-hourly TPR		1) Breathing & circulation exercises 2) Assess mobility and encourage mobilization		
Third post-op day Date Signature	1) Check wound 2) Check intestinal function 3) Assess mobility 4) Check suitability for discharge 5) Check patient understands meaning of Cholecystectomy	1) Encourage self-care 2) Check wound 3) Check TPR 4) TTO's 5) Confirm transport & district nurse 6) Discharge time		Breathing & circulation exercises	Post-op visit	
Fourth post-op day Date Signature						1) Up.ad.lib. 2) Self caring 3) Check wound 4) Post-op Education

Acute unit collaborative care plan for Cholecystectomy – audit report

Name: Reg. No: Consultant   Sex: Male/Female

Date of Admission: /   /   Primary Carers at Home:

Date of Discharge:

Outcome of objectives	Achieved	Not Achieved	Comment
Medical			
1. The patient will be admitted to hospital on the planned admission day			
2. Prior to theatre the patient and family will have had the opportunity to discuss their surgery, care and possible risks with the multidisciplinary team as appropriate			
3. In relation to the care plan the physical and psychological needs of the patient will be met			
4. The patient will be medically fit for discharge on the third post-operative day			
Nursing			
5. The patient will have attended a preadmission clinic			
6. All post operative equipment will have been checked and prepared ready for use			
7. The patient will have had the need for pain relief considered and met			
8. By discharge the patient will understand the process of wound healing, possible complications and the action to take			
9. By discharge the patient will have followed the investigatory plan			
10. The patient documentation will be completed according to the hospital policy			
11. The patient will have had the information booklet fully explained to them			
Physiotherapy			
12. Prior to theatre the patient will demonstrate breathing, circulatory and supported coughing exercises			
Theatre staff			
13. The patient will have had a pre-post operative visit			
Dietary			
14. The patient will receive dietary advice			

Coventry Community Care Unit
Collaborative care plan for cholecystectomy

Name: _____ No: _____ Discharge Date: _____

Address: _____ D.o.B. _____ GP _____

_____ Consultant: _____

Post-operative day	DNS	Patient	General practitioner	Social services

1st visit (Day after discharge)	1) Introduction to patient
	2) Assessment as per registration form
	3) Evaluate wound.
	  i) Discuss with patient
	  ii) Prepare Care Plan with patient
	  iii) apply dressing if needed. Instruct patient in dressing technique.
	
	4) Suture – evaluate – discuss with patient. Make arrangements for 10th day post-op
	  i) CNS to de-suture
	  ii) De-suture at GPs – Practice nurse
	  iii) De-suture by DNS at Health Centre
	5) Assess pain level – advice re: pain control & enhance levels of general comfort
	6) Assess – Give advice re:
	  i) Mobilisation
	  ii) Posture
	  iii) re-iterate to continue physiotherapy
	7) Diet – advise re: maintaining adequate diet & fluids
	8) Advise re: bowel activity
		3) i) Report any change in wound over last 24 hrs – oozing, pain present.
		  ii) Daily bath as able – maintain personal hygiene
		  iii) Apply dressing as instructed by DNS if needed
		4) Inform DNS of any change in suture
		
		5) Inform DNS of level of pain, any change in pain levels. Take medication as prescribed
		6) i) increasing mobilisation as able
		  ii) maintain good posture
		  iii) continue physio-therapy
		   – deep breathing
		   – supportive coughing
		7) Maintain adequate diet & fluids. Inform DNS, any problems arising
		8) Inform DNS, any change in bowel
			GP informed of patient discharge
			
			Liaise. Inform of any problems
			
			Inform surgery Practice nurse re: de-suture
			
			Liaise. Inform GP of any problems presenting
			
			Inform GP any signs, symptoms presenting
			
			Inform GP any problems arising
			
			Inform GP any problems	

Coventry Community Care Unit
Collaborative care plan for cholecystectomy

Name: _____ No: _____ Discharge Date: _____

Address: _____ D.o.B. _____ GP _____

_____   Consultant: _____

Post-operative day	DNS	Patient	General practitioner	Social services
1st visit (Day after discharge)	9) Arrange with patient date of next visit	9) i) Aware of contact numbers ii) Contact GP if needed iii) Demonstrate knowledge of condition, confident to respond to problems arising		
2nd Visit (as arranged)	1) i) Evaluate general condition ii) Evaluate wound iii) Evaluate pain level iv) Evaluate diet fluid intake v) Evaluate bowel activity vi) Evaluate mobilisation	1) Report to DNS any change or any problems present re: i) wound ii) pain level iii) diet fluid take iv) bowel activity v) mobilisation	Inform GP any problems presenting	
10th Day Post-Op	1) Evaluate general condition Evaluate wound – discuss & explain suture removal if wound satisfactory 2) Discharge patient if condition satisfactory Complete Outcome Objective Form and forward to: Mrs M. R. Mitchell, Community Liaison Sister H2, Phase IV, Walsgrave Hospital.	1) Report any problems presenting Demonstrate able to respond to problems arising and take appropriate action		

Coventry Community Care Unit

Collaborative care plan audit for Cholecystectomy patients

	Yes	No	Why	Percent
1. Were all patients over 65 years old seen at pre-admission clinic				
2. Was the patient's documentation completed according to the community nursing service policy				
3. Did the patient receive advice as nursing care plan				
4. Did the patient have the need for pain relief considered and met				
5. By discharge had the patient followed the collaborative care plan and been de-sutured on the 10th day where achievable				
6. Did the patient reach the expected level of recovery to be discharged by district nursing service on the 10th day				
7. By discharge did the patient understand the recovery period and possible complications which may arise and what actions to take				
8. By discharge did the patient feel confident that physical and psychological needs had been met where achievable				

Appendix 4   Case Management: Myocardial Infarction

Addenbrooke's NHS Trust

Addenbrooke's NHS Trust

Case Management:

Myocardial Infarction

Name:

Hosp. No.:

Consultant:

Care map	Day 1 CCU	Day 2	Day 3	Day 4	Day 5	Day 6	Day 7
Date							
Time							
Consultations	Medical Team RGN	Cardiology Ward RGN prior to transfer	Cardiac rehab therapist RGN	Cardiac rehab therapist	Dietician if:- Cholesterol ≥ 5.2 Diabetic Overweight	Physiotherapist	
Tests	ECG prn CX R U+E's/C.E.s Lipids/FBC Fluid chart O₂ Saturation Cardiac monitor V signs 1/4°–4°	ECG prn U + Es C.E.s Fluid chart Cardiac monitor 1°–4°	ECG Weight Vital signs TDS	Weight Vital signs TDS	Weight Vital signs BD	Stairs test Weight Vital signs OD	Weight
Treatments	O2 prn IV access x2	Venflon OUT on transfer to ward if not required for further treatments					

Medications	Assess for Thrombolysis Aspirin IV nitrates prn analgesia prn diuretics prn	Assess for Beta-blockers					TTOs for 7 days to include GTN
Diet	As tolerated low Fat	Low fat	Low fat	Low fat	Low fat	Low fat	Low fat
Activity	Complete bed rest. Bed pan/ commode. Bedbath/ assisted wash.	Bed rest / commode. Sit up to 1 hour twice daily.	Bed rest. Sit up to 2 hours BD. Wheel to toilet	Frequency of: Sitting Short Walks Up to toilet Wheel to bath/ Shower with help.	Walk round bay area. Frequent rest periods. Independent wash/assisted bath.	Walk freely. Independent self care. Frequent rest periods.	Fully Independent.
Teaching	Orientate to CCU. Pain Scale. Breathing & Leg exercises. Diagnosis.	Booklet 1 "Coping with Chest Pain" Risk factors Convalescence	Booklet 2 "After a Heart Attack What Now?"	DISCUSSION Patient/partner: Activity levels chest pain home/work	REINFORCE previous advice	REINFORCE previous advice	CONFIRMED CHOLESTEROL LEVEL ☐
Discharge Planning	Initial Assessment.	Preparation for transfer to ward (discontinue cardiac monitor if appropriate)	Enter patient into Cardiac Rehab. register. Assess for Social Services.			O.P. Appt. Stress test appt. ≤ 70 years	Discharge. Summary. GP letter. Provide drug info. sheets.
Signature							
Position							

Nursing care plan: myocardial infarction

Activity problem/need	Goal	Day 1	Day 2
1. Teaching knowledge deficit	Patient and family have increased knowledge of I.H.D.	Identify Risk factors and explain aetiology of MI	Patient will participate in individual teaching plan.
2. Emotional Support anxiety	Patient and family will feel supported	Explain Rationale for CCU Patient and family will feel able to express their anxieties.	Assess family Support Systems
3. Pain potential for ischaemic pain	Patient states pain scale 0	Instruct patient to state if any chest pain/discomfort Teach pain scale Monitor severity and record chest pain. Define nature of chest pain	
4. Nutrition potential risk factors from diet	i. Understand rationale for low fat diet. ii. Patient will be motivated to eat low fat diet.	Provide low fat diet as tolerated. Observe dietary intake	
5. Elimination i. potential for low urine output ii. potential for constipation.	Patient will perform normal daily elimination process. Record abnormalities of urinalysis.	Accurate fluid balance chart. Inform Dr if BP ↓ & anuric.	Record bowel function. Fluid balance chart.
6. Hygiene inability to maintain normal hygiene pattern.	Patient should be as independent as condition allows.	Bed bath (with assistance). Hands and face wash PRN.	
7. Observations potential arrhythmias and altered haemodynamic status	Sinus rhythm rate < 100 BP ↑100 systolic Patient warm and well perfused.	Cardiac monitor 1/4°–1° BP+P. 1° BP+P 4° BP+P 4° Temp Oxygen sat PRN	1°–4° BP+P 4° Temp
8. Mobilisation enforced limited mobility	Patient will be able to maintain activity level without problems.	Assess and evaluate patient's progress. Inform Dr of any complications.	
9. Respiration potential dyspnoea due to myocardial damage.	Resp. rate < 24 O2 sat > 95% HR < 100 Wt stable.	Record resp rate 1°–4° Record oxygen sats PRN Fluid balance.	
10. Safety environment i. potential side effects of SK infusion within 24 hrs ii Potential for unsuitable home environment	i. No major:- haemorrhage. haematoma formation anaphylaxis, hypotension ii. Home environment suitable for discharge.	i. SK obs if appropriate Observe for phlebitis Patency of IV cannula ii. Assess whether carers at home are available.	
Other Problems	See Separate Care plan		
Signatures AM			
PM			
Nocte			

Day 3	Day 4	Day 5	Day 6	Day 7
Orientation to wards	Assess patient's knowledge of the risk factors of IHD.	Assess knowledge about dealing with chest pain. Identify any knowledge deficits. Reinforce advice in Booklet I & II.		Advise about medication.
Identify potential problems or worries. Support Patient + Family.				
12 lead ECG Provide Nitrates if BP allows/analgesia prn If persistent pain or ECG changes inform Dr.				
Record bowel function.				
SEE CARE MAP				
SEE CARE MAP Observe for side effect of medication and report to Dr.				
Assess and evaluate patient's progress. Inform Dr. of any complications.				
SEE CARE MAP				
ii Check social services have been contacted.	ii Ensure relatives feel confident and supported.			

Name:

Hosp. No.:

Consultant:

	Date of Admission	Date of Discharge

Date	Variances (please tick)	Variance code	State reason if not covered by code

Medical

_____	Lipids not taken	☐	_____
_____	Thrombolysis/Aspirin not given	☐	_____
_____	IV Heparin given	☐	_____
_____	Nitrates not given	☐	_____
_____	Day 2 Bloods not taken	☐	_____

Nursing

_____	< or > 24 hour stay CCU	☐	_____
_____	ECG not taken Day 2	☐	_____
_____	Day 3	☐	_____
_____	Day 7	☐	_____
_____	Different regime for activity level	☐	_____
_____	Drug information sheets not given	☐	_____
_____	TTO (including GTN) for 7 days not ordered prior to discharge	☐	_____
_____	OPA & Stress Test Appointment not made	☐	_____
_____	Reason for longer stay than 7 days	☐	_____
_____	Reason for coming off Case Management system	☐	_____

Rehab

_____	Cardiac Rehab Therapist ┐	☐	_____
_____	Physiotherapist ├ no visit	☐	_____
_____	Dietician ┘	☐	_____

_____	Other _____	☐	_____
_____	Other _____	☐	_____

1. Overlooked	5. Not required	9. No beds on CCU
2. Patient's general condition	6. Contra-indicated	10. Enzymes not raised
3. Arrhythmias	7. Duration of pain	11. Social circumstances
4. Chest pain	8. No beds on medical unit	

Variance coding

Index